HOSPITAL ADMINISTRATION FROM THE PERSPECTIVE OF NON-MEDICAL EXECUTIVES - THE UNSUNG HEROES

VISHWA BANDHU JOSHI
WITH A FOREWORD BY DR. MAHESH SHARMA

BlueRose
Publishers
NewDelhi • London

First Published in December 2021

ISBN: 978-93-5472-946-1

BLUEROSE PUBLISHERS
www.bluerosepublishers.com
info@bluerosepublishers.com
+91 8882 898 898

Cover Design:
Geetika

Typographic Design:
Namrata Saini

Distributed by: BlueRose, Amazon, Flipkart, Shopclues

डा महेश शर्मा

सांसद–लोक सभा गौतमबुद्धनगर, उ.प्र.

Dr. Mahesh Sharma
Member of Parliament - Lok Sabha
Gautam Budh Nagar, U.P.

पूर्व राज्यमंत्री पर्यटन एवं संस्कृति (स्वतंत्र प्रभार),
नागरिक उड्डयन, वन एवं पर्यावरण राज्यमंत्री,
भारत सरकार

Former Minister of State (I/C) Tourism & Culture,
Minister of State for Civil Aviation, Environment
& Forest, Govt. of India

Date : 24.07.2021

Foreword

The healthcare sector runs with the synergetic efforts of both medicos and non-medicos, who complement each other to meet the objective of the sector – to provide care to patients successfully and satisfactorily. While the medicos treat the patients, it is the non-medicos who enable them to do so, predominantly by working behind the scenes. Therefore, the critical role that the non-medicos play often gets overshadowed by the work medicos do. In his book — **"Hospital Administration from the Perspective of Non-Medical Executives – the Unsung Heroes"** — Mr Vishwa Bandhu Joshi, who has been with Kailash Healthcare Limited as a non-medical executive for over 20 years, has highlighted the roles the non-medicos play and the challenges they face. Not only that, using his vast experience in the healthcare sector as a non-medico, he has given several advice and suggestions for policymakers and curriculum formulators in hospital administration.

Dr. Mahesh Sharma

Camp Office : H-33, Sector-27, Noida-201 301 • Tel.: 0120-244 44 44, 246 66 66 • Fax : 0120-254 44 88
Delhi Office : 13, Talkatora Road, New Delhi - 110 001 • Tel.: 011-2331 1266 • Telefax: 011-2331 1366
Mobile : 9873444255 • E-mail : drmahesh3333@gmail.com • Website : www.drmaheshsharma.com

Inspiration

In the epic Ramayana, Lord Hanuman demonstrated all the qualities required to manage a complex medical emergency when Lord Ram's younger brother, Lakshman, was seriously injured during his battle with Lanka's King Ravan's eldest son, Meghnad. Lakshman could be saved by only one herb – the **Sanjivanibooti**. He took a giant leap from Lanka to Mount Dronagiri or Gandhamardhan hills, far to the north of the Vindhyas – on the slopes of the Himalayas. Unable to identify the life-saving herb, he moved the mountain on his shoulder and carried it to the battlefield where Lakshman was all but dead. And the rest is history.

This book is an effort to highlight how non-medical staff in a hospital move mountains round the clock, every day, day in and day out, to save the lives of patients.

I dedicate this book to the non-medical executives in hospitals – the unsung heroes of our healthcare system.

Gurudakshina

This book is dedicated to the relentless efforts of non-medical staff, who shoulder crucial responsibilities in running hospitals. The revenue generated from this book will go for the welfare of those unsung heroes and their families.

A thought for hospital planners

On an average 65 per cent to 70 per cent of non-medicos (administrators, managers, supervisors, pharmacists, nurses, paramedical staff, ward boys, clerks, housekeeping staff, etc) support 30 per cent to 35 per cent of the medicos (doctors, dentists, physiotherapists) for best medical treatment to produce the best results. However, when doctors get all the accolades, like recognitions in the form of awards and rewards, the support staff, who play a critical role in the doctors' achievements, are overlooked.

This is particularly true for India where there are countless doctors who have been conferred upon prestigious national awards, like the Padma awards, no non-medical staff has got such recognition until now.

This book seeks to highlight some of the critical roles the non-medicos play in the operation of hospitals, whose contribution in the healthcare sector must also be recognized.

"They are the unsung heroes behind the heroes." – VBJ

This book is divided into two parts:

Part I discusses the various hospital departments and the problems they face.

Part II elaborates with examples and case studies, including imaginative ones, how a hospital administrator deals with solving the problems discussed in the first part and the challenges he faces to resolve them.

About the author:

The author is an administrator in one of the best-known super-multispeciality hospitals in India. He has more than 20 years of first-hand experience in the healthcare sector as a non-medical professional.

Contents

PART – I 1

Preface 3

Lesson 1 Introduction 5

Lesson 2 The Hospital 7

Lesson 3 Administration department 15

Lesson 4 Administrator's role in casualty/emergency department 20

Lesson 5 Outpatient, preventive check-up and physiotherapy department (OPD) 38

Lesson 6 Intensive care unit (ICU) 45

Lesson 7 Operation theatre (OT) 49

Lesson 8 Wards 52

Lesson 9 Nursing department 57

Lesson 10 Laboratories & diagnostics department 61

Lesson 11 Blood bank department 65

Lesson 12 Central sterile supply department 67

Lesson 13 Admission and billing department 70

Lesson 14 Third-party administration (TPA) department 75

Lesson 15 Accounts, finance, secretarial and legal departments 79

Lesson 16 Store and pharmacy 83

Lesson 17 Information technology (IT) department 86

Lesson 18 Medical records department (MRD) 88

Lesson 19 Kitchen department 90

Lesson 20 Housekeeping department 93

Lesson 21 Laundry department 98

Lesson 22 Horticulture department 100

Lesson 23 Security and parking department 102

Lesson 24 Transport department 108

Lesson 25 Maintenance and biomedical department 112

Lesson 26 Reception department 116

Lesson 27 Marketing department... 118

Lesson 28 Quality department 121

Lesson 29 Feedback panel... 123

Lesson 30 Personnel/Human resource department 125

PART – II From the administrator's desk................................... 129

Lesson 1 Safeguarding hospital's interests...................................... 131

Lesson 2 Tackling unexpected issues 136

Lesson 3 Small things matter... 141

Lesson 3A Home collection of samples 144

Lesson 3B Maintenance department issues 146

Lesson 3C Billing complaints... 148

Lesson 4 Media and healthcare sector... 151

Lesson 4A Importance of keeping focus on work 155

Lesson 4B Patient dissatisfaction, psychology of patient
and attendants 158

Lesson 4C Administrative challenges for VVIP/VIP/general
patients 161

Lesson 5 Handling everyday problems in the ICU and ward 164

Lesson 5A Challenges during Covid-19 pandemic........................... 168

Lesson 5B Issues with communication and public relations 179

Lesson 5C Importance of training and boosting the confidence of
housekeeping staff... 182

Lesson 6 Final words from the hospital administrator 185

References 188

Acknowledgement 189

Glossary 191

PART – I

Preface

Freshmen who just joined as administrators in a hospital after completing their hospital management courses lack practical experience in handling routine functioning of hospitals. Although this is relevant in many other professions, it is particularly glaring in the healthcare industry. Unlike other industries, the healthcare industry is quite different since it deals with the life and death of human beings. Therefore, there is a need to codify the treatment and care processes.

Keeping this in mind, I have decided to write this book on hospital administration. The theme of the book is "the pride of a hospital administrator". It will have all the minute details. An aspiring new hospital administrator can get the idea of administrative issues and understand that there is no such thing as a "problem". It is just the "absence of an idea to find a solution".

This book hopes that it can inspire aspiring young administrators who join the healthcare industry and perform their duties professionally.

This book seeks to share a glimpse of the administrative achievements while working as an "unsung hero".

I have not named any particular hospital administrator, specific dates of incidents, names of the patients, staff, etc, to respect their privacy as well as the ethical codes that govern the healthcare industry.

The idea is to focus on administrative jobs and responsibilities with practical personal experiences one is expected to encounter through case studies.

Staff dealing with patients must go beyond rules to help them. This would strengthen the relationship and trust between the service provider and the ailing community.

I am grateful to my mentor Sri RN Sharma, my parents, and my family who have motivated me to write on this subject.

I am also a non-medical hospital executive and look forward to suggestions from the readers. This would help me to include some of them in the second edition of this book. — *Vishwa Bandhu Joshi*

Lesson 1

Introduction

Healthcare is the world's largest industry. To meet challenges in this sector, which keeps on changing with time and upgradation of knowledge in the field of science and technology, and medical management courses, a smart administrator is always on demand.

The hospital administration department handles day-to-day operations effectively and efficiently in running the hospitals. This is the only department that handles and controls patients and employees – directly or indirectly. It is also responsible to a great extent for the satisfaction of both patients as well as employees. Therefore, the administration always plays the most significant role in the growth of the hospitals.

In hospitals, the key input comes from the patients/patients' attendants. And other inputs come from hospital employees, including medical and non-medical staff. The administration handles all key problems of the hospital without disturbing the facility's basic constitution. Therefore, the administrator is flexible and changes its gear as the situation demands and controls all problems.

To summarize: Hospital administration is a unique profession in the healthcare industry that handles and controls the smooth functioning of routine hospital services, without hampering its operation. The administration department handles the manpower, money and machine and method directly or indirectly. In the process, it helps in providing quality care to patients as well as safeguarding the employees and the interests of the hospitals.

"Hospital administration handles all key problems of hospitals without disturbing the constitution of the facility. Hospital administrators are flexible and change their gear as the situation demands." – VBJ

History

Earlier, doctors used to assign compounder-paramedical or their personal staff to handle day-to-day activities. However, in late the 1970's, due to the rising number of private clinics, nursing homes and private hospitals, doctors started managing their administration with their friends or relatives, sometimes with the help of hired retired defence personnel or former corporate executives as "multitasking" caretakers or administrators. In those days, administrators were underpaid and their working hours were indefinite.

During those times, the so-called administrators used to apply their common sense in carrying out their duties. At times, doctors simply appointed a college graduate or even a non-graduate to play this vital role despite being grossly untrained to work as an administrator. Apart from being under par to carry out their job as an administrator in caregiving facilities, the so-called administrators used to be in touch with the police, media, and other influential people to cover their backs should a mishap happen while they performed their duties.

This is a tell-tale sign of their lack of confidence in their own job! A job that they volunteered to undertake. In the slightest instance of "mishandling" a situation, they ran to the concerned hospital's management. It reflected the fact that such administrators never went to the root cause of the problems but worked only when a problem presented itself.

Things started to change in the late 1980s and 1990s when universities started courses in hospital management. That was the time when hospitals started getting "corporatized".

Hospitals started appointing fresh university graduates armed with a degree in hospital management.

However, there was a catch!

Even in these graduation courses, the students were taught more on medicine and management courses with key focus on corporate management only and not on hardcore administration.

Every hospital – private, corporate, government – however big or small, has different job requirements and responsibilities for the administrator. Hence the key responsibilities areas are to liaison, coordinate, and implement policies framed by hospital management for smooth functioning of care giving facilities.

Lesson 2

The Hospital

A hospital is a place where people come for clinical diagnosis, advice for medication, therapeutic counselling, and treatment for all kinds of sickness, injuries and any mental or physical health suffering. The hospital works around the clock throughout the year, and is involved with a person right from birth to his end of life – death.

Operational shifts

A hospital provides service around the clock throughout the year. Therefore, shift duty in the healthcare industry is inevitable. However, handing over or taking over charges, especially by doctors, nurses, paramedics, floor managers, ward boys/*aya*, housekeeping staff, etc, should be transparent so that no lapses can happen due to miscommunication. Sometimes, due to the casual approach in taking charges, major problems emerge and even risk of life can happen (in rare cases). In such a situation, the medical superintendent or the administrator or sometimes authorities from the higher step in resolving the issue as the goodwill of the hospital is at stake. Hence, after each shift, proper handing/taking over charge should be done with written documentation duly signed by both the incoming and the outgoing staff and the same should be kept in a file to avoid lapses. An early appearance of 10–15 minutes before shift time is expected for each staff so that the changeover is seamless.

In some NABH (National Accreditation Board for Hospitals and Healthcare Providers)-accredited hospitals, ISBAR (Identify, Situation, Background, Assessment & Recommendation) concept is used. It is a mnemonic created to improve safety in the transfer of critical information at each level of staff working in different departments.

Even the floor manager, ward manager, and the administrator must follow the same and understand, that is, prognosis/treatmentpayment status cash/through panel/MLC etc. So that whole could be controlled and managed by the next shift administrator.

Typically, a hospital has three operational shifts:

1. Morning
2. Evening
3. Night

The medical superintendent controls the hospital, the chief administrator controls the non-medical staff, and the nursing superintendent controls the nursing staff. In some hospitals, the management/owner appoints a chief executive officer who is tasked with running the facility.

The hospital's medical superintendent, chief administrator and nursing superintendent make the rules for their subordinates and delegate power to them for successfully running the facility.

Of late, a trend has been seen in hospitals where the management gives designation to people, like president, vice-president, group director, director, etc, according to their convenience and requirement. A majority of those who hold these posts are doctors or chartered accountants/company secretaries/ lawyers or those who have experience in management. They help the organization in a range of things, like diversification, expansion, development. They also take part in policymaking.

Morning shift:

The operations department working in morning and general shift are as follows:

1. Casualty department: It runs round the clock every day of the year.
2. Outpatient and preventive check-up departments: They run in morning and evening every day.
3. Wards, day care, intensive care units, operation theatres, and dialysis units: They run round the clock each day of the year.
4. Nursing department: It runs round the clock every day of the year.
5. Lab & diagnostic centre: It runs round the clock every day of the year.
6. Pharmacy: It runs round the clock every day of the year.
7. Central sterile supply department: It runs round the clock every day of the year.
8. Transport (ambulances and hearse vans): It runs around the clock every day of the year.

9. Security and parking department: It runs around the clock every day of the year.
10. Housekeeping department: It runs around the clock every day of the year.
11. Laundry department: It runs around the clock every day of the year.
12. Information technology (IT) department
13. Maintenance department: It runs around the clock every day of the year.
14. Blood bank: It runs around the clock all throughout the year.
15. Reception: It runs round the clock every day of the year.
16. Kitchen department
17. Marketing department
18. Accounts, finance, secretarial, and legal departments
19. TPA department
20. Medical record department
21. HR department
22. Quality department
23. Horticulture department

The medical superintendent, chief administrator and nursing superintendent don't interfere in day-to-day operations of the accounts, finance, HR, IT, marketing, quality, and other departments. However, if they face any problem pertaining to the abovementioned departments, only then they interact in the interest of patient care.

A person who has experience and exposure to human resources management controls the HR department. The heads of the departments of accounts, finance, company secretary and the legal advisor are well qualified in their field of specialization and are known as non-medicos. They run their departments and report to the owners or the top management of the hospital.

Evening shift:

The evening operations of hospital services start from 3pm to 9pm depending upon the season. During this shift, meetings of the management/board of directors usually take place.

The evening shift has the following operational departments:

1. Causality/Admission/Reception
2. OPD/Day care
3. Minor OT/OT/Procedure
4. Dental
5. Physiotherapy
6. Internal ward
7. ICU
8. Dialysis department
9. Lab & diagnostic/Non-invasive services
10. Pharmacy
11. IT
12. Parking and security
13. Housekeeping
14. Third-party administrator, who fixes problems related to the health insurance claims.
15. Blood bank.
16. Maintenance Department.
17. Kitchen

Night shift:

In this shift, security plays a very vital role, which includes guarding the building, patients and staff from any unforeseen security threat. This is a critical shift as most of the patients who come to a hospital at night need emergency care.

"The causality services take care of the entire load of hospitals. The causality department transforms into a mini hospital at night." - VBJ

The following departments remain closed during the night shift:

1. OPD.
2. HR department.
3. Accounts department.

4. Company secretarial department.

5. Advertisement/Marketing department.

6. Medical records department.

7. Quality control department.

8. Non-invasive services department.

9. Preventive check-up department.

10. Horticulture department.

11. Kitchen (Partially open for only emergency services for ICU, ward, neonatal, paediatric intensive care unit).

In short, the night shift operates mainly with the following departments:

1. Emergency department.

2. Admission/Billing department.

3. ICU.

4. Ward.

5. Lab & diagnostic/CSSD/Laundry department.

6. OT.

7. Dialysis.

8. Reception.

9. IT.

10. Security/Parking.

11. Maintenance department.

12. Housekeeping department.

13. Pharmacy department.

14. Blood bank.

A majority of hospitals have night managers, sister (nurse) in charge, chief casualty medical officers to run their night services.

A hospital works like a power backup system, which means all three shifts – under the three people in charge or supervisors – enable the hospital to render its services seamlessly.

The idea for keeping supervisor and staff in three shifts are as follows:

1. The entire team is agile, alert and competent.

2. Routine powers of execution remain with the in charge or supervisor, which gives more freedom and confidence to the shift in charge to take decisions in the interest of patient care.

3. The in charge takes care of almost all the issues without disturbing the management or hospital authority during the night shift. However, if there is any unforeseen incident, the night managers inform their seniors about it. After getting the information, the medical superintendent/ administrator/ management staff comes to the hospital to lead from the front in reputed hospitals.

The institution is more important than the individual. If any senior executive leaves the hospital, then there is hardly any vacuum in the leadership hierarchy. The management always ensures that there is a backup plan for such contingencies.

In the absence of the three-tier system as discussed, it has been observed that the medical superintendent, chief administrator, and nursing superintendent get calls from hospitals even for minor issues at odd hours. This has resulted in health issues for them in the long run. It also distressed their families. Too much workload and the pressure that comes along with it affects the quality of their work. Apart from this, their family lives also get affected.

This is the sole reason why hospitals maintain three shifts and deploy a three-tier chain of command.

A hospital has two categories of employees:

1. Medicos

2. Non-medicos

Medicos

Countless books are published for doctors, dentists and physiotherapists by medical researchers, academics, renowned doctors, etc. These books contain a treasure of knowledge gained by doctors. There are several fellowship programmes regarding the treatment of patients.

Doctors, dentists and physiotherapists also attend seminars, conferences and other programmes every now and then to upgrade their caregiving and treatment skills. Top bodies for doctors, like the Indian Medical Association and state medical associations safeguard the interests of the doctor fraternity. Even students studying medicine have resident doctors' associations, who safeguard their interests.

Even the central and state governments hear their grievances from time to time.

Non-medicos

In every hospital, non-medicos are of all levels. They are the housekeeping staff, laundry staff, security staff, kitchen staff, ward boys, woman helpers (*ayas*), waiters, paramedical, technicians, drivers, transport and ambulance services staff, maintenance staff, accountants, marketing staff, legal advisers, company secretaries, pharmacists, nursing staff, radiology technicians, etc.

Without their help and support, the doctors would fail to give care or treat a patient and the hospital's main reason to exist would fail.

Most of the non-medical staff come from villages or small towns. A good number of them are those who come to cities or towns seeking jobs. Most of them who join the healthcare sector as non-medicos are not driven by the noble cause to serve but to make a living. An overwhelming majority of them start liking their job and remain in the healthcare sector throughout their service life – constantly learning new skills while serving the healthcare sector and society at large. While working as non-medical staff in hospitals, many of them learn great professional skills. Several of them have reached higher levels, like supervisors, paramedical, technicians and even managers despite not having formal qualification in the field.

In other words, the non-medico employees are composed of a mixture of unskilled, skilled, uneducated, and educated workers. They have four sets of classes.

1. The employees who are educated up to Class X work as housekeepers, labourers, security guards, peons, or assigned to do multiple tasks.

2. Those who have had formal school education from Class X to XII work as drivers, ward boys, *ayas*, Assistant, etc.

3. The employees who have relevant diplomas, work as technicians, paramedical, computer operators, electricians, etc.

4. Those who are graduates and postgraduates with university degrees, like BA, BCom, MA, MCom, MSc, MBA or are qualified BPharmas, MPharmas, Bachelors in Hospital Administration, Masters in Hospital Administration, BSc in Nutrition and Dietetics, CAs, CSs, data-entry

operators, etc, are employed in the accounts, finance, company secretarial, pharmacy, and kitchen departments.

New trends in hospitals

Nowadays, doctors refer their patients to other specialists for being doubly sure about their diagnosis for further treatment and illness management. Due to this, patients directly or through their attendants are advised to carry out tests recommended by specialists for detailed investigations for diagnosis and treatment. This has become a routine practice in almost all multispecialty hospitals.

The non-medicos ensure the above process and coordinate with the patients right from the time they enter the hospital until they leave. During the time in between the patient's entry and exist, the non-medicos run pillar to post to arrange things, like timely meeting with treating doctor/referral consultant, laboratories/diagnostic test, make arrangements for procedures, if needed. They also assist in other issues, like parking, registration, appointment, billing, TPA pharmacy, kitchen service, etc.

"The non-medicos is the lifeline that enables a hospital to render its services and supports doctors to treat patients. They are the railroad that the train of the hospital runs on." – VBJ

Lesson 3

Administration department

In the healthcare sector, there are many departments, like accounting, physiotherapy, finance, pathology, radiology, and many more. However, each of these departments is ultimately controlled, either directly or indirectly by the administration department, which dictates all policies.

The administration department is one of the main authorities of a hospital, and it is its duty to manage, control and delegate the various responsibilities to the appropriate people. The administration department is a crucial part of the hospital, which deals with the social, economic, legal and political aspects of running the organization. They don't involve themselves in medical treatment.

Each hospital has a chief administrator, whose responsibility is to oversee and organize everything, ensuring that the hospital runs smoothly, unhampered by any administrative issues.

The hospital administrator is the one who plans and dictates policy, balancing the needs and resources of the hospital to optimize the hospital's functions. The administrator should ideally administer the hospital's sphere of activities in a holistic way, with a clear chain of command and defined authority. There should be rules and protocols concerning the delegation of authority and responsibility, as well as clear lines of communication between all the hospital departments to avoid ambiguity and maximize efficiency.

Qualifications and traits of an administrator

The crucial skills and abilities that a competent hospital administrator must possess are:

1. They must have either a graduate degree or a postgraduate degree, and in both cases, they must also have considerable experience working at a hospital.

2. Well-developed social skills and good health.

3. There should be a good understanding of the business and administration of a hospital, so that they know who to talk during various issues and concern.

4. The patients' interests should be their priority, and they should be proactive in solving problems, such as taking the initiative to reach out to patients and patient attendants to obtain a firm grasp of their issues and how to solve them.

5. The ability to remain calm and focused in a crisis, and to avoid becoming complacent.

6. A checklist for the various departments and areas, to make sure everything is running smoothly and to mitigate any problems.

7. A list of contingency plans for crisis situations, which should all be carefully designed to balance the needs and desires of the patients, customers and employees while still being in line with hospital policy.

8. A willingness to examine each problem in-depth, so as to root out the cause and prevent it from happening again.

9. The administrator must take the initiative to tackle the problems directly instead of off-loading their responsibilities on their subordinates, who may lack the knowledge and authority to deal with issues properly.

Let me give you two examples to highlight how this can be useful:

Case 1

Once, a middle-aged person came to the hospital at 7pm with his daughter, who had suffered a traumatic foot injury. The doctor suggested an x-ray should be taken of the daughter's injured leg, and the man paid for it. However, the man was a CGHS beneficiary, and requested the doctor to write "emergency" in the prescription so that he could be reimbursed by his office. The doctor refused, and so did the casualty manager. This led to a heated argument between the two sides for 2–3 hours. Thus, a minor issue became a major problem which was not resolved until the hospital administrator was called in. The administrator apologized for the delay and discussed the issue with the hospital's chief casualty medical officer (CCMO). The CCMO then advised the doctor to write the word "emergency" on the prescription, at which point the man paid for his daughter's treatment and happily left.

*[**Note:** The administrator didn't directly ask/advise the treating doctor to write the word "emergency" on the prescription, but took the issue to the chief CMO, who then did the needful, respecting the hierarchy.]*

The administrator made a point to stay in touch with the man over the next two months and checked to make sure that the man was refunded. Once the man was refunded the money that he had paid for his daughter's treatment, he thanked the administrator, and he and his family became regular visitors to the hospital whenever they faced any health issue.

Case 2

An aged patient suffering from a chronic obstructive pulmonary disease (COPD), was admitted to a single room, where there was an excessive amount of sound from a nearby construction site. The patient's daughter was angered, and complained to the reception and the night manager, but they said they could not solve the problem as the construction site was right next door to the hospital. Frustrated, the patient's daughter asked to speak to the administrator, who was called. The administrator listened to her grievances, contacted the construction site and with the aid of the night security officers, persuaded them to halt construction for the night. The night manager could have solved the issue himself if he had been more proactive, but in the end, the chief administrator had to intervene himself to resolve the issue.

10. A wise administrator should keep a suggestion register in each ward pertaining to the issues that patients and their attendants face. This helps the administrator to remain informed and allows him to swiftly intervene in any problematic situations.

*[**Note:** Most hospitals give a feedback form at the time of discharge to the patient or the patient's attendant. Then the filled form is dropped in the suggestion box. The suggestion box is opened once every fifteen days or once a month depending on hospital policy. The suggestions are reviewed by a committee where the administrator is also a key member of the committee.]*

11. Administrators must develop mechanisms to assess the gravity of a problematic situation and focus on solving it as swiftly as possible, rather than providing a post facto solution.

12. They should be able to maintain good relations with outside organizations such as the government, media, judiciary etc.

13. The administrator must have a firm grasp of IT, computer language, sign language and code.

14. They should not allow their ego and personal feelings to interfere with their work, and be able to put them aside to work towards the best interests of the hospital.

15. A wise administrator always works towards solving issues rather than explaining or narrating facts. An astute administrator should always be well informed and aware of his/her authority and duties.

16. Strategizing the solution within available resources is a key deliverable of an administrator. In layman's language don't be part of a problem or be in explanation mode. Be a part of the solution.

Words of caution:

1. An administrator is a non-medico professional, hence should not get involved in the treatment of patients.

2. The administrator must follow ethical norms while utilizing his official resources, time, and authority. He/she must not use his/her resources for personal use.

3. Don't take for granted any staff, whether senior or junior. Strictly stick to the hospital's norms.

4. During duty hours, avoid diverting your attention by doing things like talking to your colleagues, using mobiles for personal use, chatting with friends, etc. Always keep full focus on the task at hand.

5. Whenever aggrieved patients/patients' attendants enter "frustration mode", most of the times they believe that their grievances are not resolved by the hospital. During such times, the first job of the chief administrator is to pacify the aggrieved patient/attendant by showing empathy and creating a conducive environment to address the issue.

To summarize: A hospital administrator must be proactive, accountable, intelligent and well-informed. Remember, once a patient or/and his/her attendant come(s) to the hospital, they expect prompt attention as well as speedy recovery. The hospital faces an uphill task of gaining their trust with responsible and focused actions.

The administrator works as a bridge between the patient and the hospital. He/she arranges everything for the patient from admission to discharge during the patient's treatment to the best of their satisfaction.

"The administrator must connect with patients on humanitarian level, show empathy and take meaningful actions to uphold their faith reposed on the hospital by focusing on quality treatment and building trust consistently." – VBJ

Lesson 4

Administrator's role in casualty/emergency department

Emergency services are the face of the hospital. Entire set of people (medical and non-medical) work as a team to carry out the implementation/execution of standard operative procedures to treat patients.

Three classes of patients come to the emergency department:

a.   Conscious patient

b.   Unconscious patient

c.   Brought dead patient

For each class of patient, the role of staff medical/non-medical is well defined by hospital management. The standard operative procedure in most hospitals is almost the same for the emergency department. However, a key difference between ordinary hospitals and reputed hospitals are:

a.   Education, training, and experience of manpower (medical/non-medical staff).

b.   Infrastructure.

c.   Technological advancement in all areas.

Each step of patient care is well documented for doctors, nurses and all the staff working at the casualty area, that is, checklist, implementation and execution of standard Operation procedure.

The role of the administrator in casualty is to coordinate/liaison with staff on a need basis and also ensure the best medical attention to each patient coming to the emergency area.

The administrator coordinates with the following departments and staff to give best medical attention:

1. Security guards at the casualty gate.
2. Ward boys/*ayas*
3. Nurses, doctors, consultants
4. Paramedical staff
5. Laboratory & diagnostics department
6. Day care/IPD/OT
7. Blood bank and pharmacy
8. Admission file/billing department/TPA /Panel
9. Cashier
10. Maintenance
11. Housekeeping
12. Biomedical / Oxygen plant, CSSD
13. Kitchen
14. Reception
15. Laundry
16. MRD
17. Management
18. Transportation (ambulance and hearse services)
19. Miscellaneous

Duties of a security guard (stationed at the emergency gate):

1. A security guard must ensure that the process of a patient's arrival and departure are smooth. This includes directing vehicles to the parking area/exit after a patient has been dropped off, or keeping an eye on patients who are taking leave against medical advice (LAMA) and discharge on request (DOR) to go to another hospital.

2. Maintaining peace in and around the casualty area. A guard must also carefully handle aggressive patients and/or attendants if they require

extra help, as well as inform the casualty manager of any problem, who in turn will call additional security or police as required.

3. To supervise and safeguard hospital property in the casualty area.

4. Arrange safe passage for a patient who is being shifted to the ICU/ward/diagnostic area, especially one in critical condition.

5. Miscellaneous duties. Let me give you three possible scenarios:

Scenario 1:

During rush hours, a patient's attendant may hurriedly park a car near the casualty area to enable him/her to move the patient to the emergency department quicker, and take the car keys with him/her, causing issues for the security staff. In such a case, a team of security staff must remove the car to a proper place.

Scenario 2:

Once, a patient's attendant stole the mobile phone of another patient. On inquiry by the latter's attendant the security staff checked the CCTV footage and found the culprit. They called the thieving attendant and warned him that he would face consequences if he didn't return the phone. Fearing legal action, the thief returned the phone at the security gate. This proves how and why a CCTV camera system is compulsory for even a hospital, and that a casualty manager/security in charge must ensure it is functional all the time.

Scenario 3:

In rare cases, during rush hours a patient quietly takes away the case file without informing the hospital and goes missing. A watchful security guard should be able to catch hold of the patient along with the case file and bring him/her to the administrator. The administrator then asks their choice whether to stay in the hospital or leave legally. If they don't agree to stay or leave legally, the administrator, respecting their decision, discharges the patient as "leave against medical advice" (LAMA).

If any unknown patient is brought to the hospital, the casualty manager contacts security for aid in identifying the patient. If a security guard observes any person looking for the unaccompanied/unknown patient, he immediately informs the security head/casualty manager.

Some problems the administration staff can face in a casualty ward because of incompetent security staff are:

a. New guards coming to work at the casualty ward are mostly unqualified for the job, as they often lack the needed intelligence and aptitude.

b. Contractual guards, who lack knowledge of how the hospital works.

c. Frequent changing of guards, which prevents them from developing the experience and confidence they need to handle the casualty area.

d. A non-functional CCTV due to poor maintenance, which prevents evidence from being recorded.

e. Additional guards are not provided when requested.

f. A security guard who does not know how to speak properly to his colleagues or the patients, speaking loudly and aggressively, thus causing arguments and even fights.

The security staff play an important role in the hospital, and without them, an administrative manager will likely end up having to waste a lot of time in solving problems. One common problem a hospital administrator faces is while dealing with injuries and/or death caused by road-traffic accidents (RTA) or "brought dead" patients.

Sometimes, the person who hit the injured patient comes along to help, and remains until the patient's family and friends arrive. When the latter sees the person responsible for injuring the patient, it may lead to quarrels, which requires the security staff to step in. The administrative manager then must brief both parties on the hospital protocol. For example:

1. The hospital only provides treatment.

2. Disputes must be settled in the police station or court, outside of hospital premises.

3. The attendant can either continue to receive treatment here, or switch to a hospital of their choice.

4. All RTA cases require MLC.

In cases concerning death or serious injuries, sometimes the patient attendants may become stressed, angry, aggressive and start unnecessary arguments with security and administration staff. It is the duty of the casualty manager and security guards to maintain order, and if necessary, call the police for aid in safeguarding the hospital's staff and interests.

Other issues can also arise, such as financial problems when a doctor explains their prognosis to a patient attendant, or when a patient doesn't wish to continue treatment and leave as LAMA. The administrative manager must counsel the patients and if they are unwilling to listen, the manager must respect their wishes and decisions.

Suggestions:

1. Only experienced and capable security guards who understand the gravity of such situations should be assigned to the emergency department.
2. If called, the security officials must deploy aid to the emergency area swiftly and effectively.

Ward boy/*aya* at emergency area

Duties of ward boys and/or *ayas*:

1. Help to shift patients after carefully taking them off vehicles, like ambulances, to the casualty area and following the instructions of the doctors, nurses and casualty manager.
2. Help to shift patients to the investigation/Laboratory & diagnostics area.
3. Help patients to shift to ICU/OT/minor OT/day care/ward, according to the instructions of their superiors.
4. Do part preparation for patients going for surgery under the supervision of the nursing staff.

Some problems hospital administrators face when dealing with ward boys and *aya*s:

a. While being shifted, a patient falls down due to the carelessness of the ward boy/*aya* in rare cases.
b. In rare cases, sometimes valuables are stolen or go missing while the patient is being shifted. When such things happen, CCTV footage can be useful to solve the case.
c. Monitors are not in place while the patient is being shifted to the ICU/ward/diagnostic and investigation area.
d. New ward boys and *ayas* are assigned without training.

e. When a patient is being taken off from an ambulance, oxygen cylinders/monitors are not kept in place. One common problem that ward boys/*ayas* face is when a patient forgets where he/she placed his/her footwear in the casualty area. The duty ward boy/*aya* must put the footwear in a bag or hand it to their attendant. If an attendant is not available, they should put it in a cupboard/rack meant for keeping patient's items.

Word of caution:

In case of gunshot wounds or medicolegal cases, the casualty manager must preserve the patient's clothes and every other belonging in a sealed bag for future legal purposes.

Observations:

1. A ward boy is required to check all equipment with the aid of paramedics and nurses. If there is any deficient or damaged equipment, it must be replaced or repaired. For example, wheelchairs, stretchers, oxygen cylinders and monitors should all be carefully inspected before a patient is shifted to another area of the hospital.

2. A trained ward boy/*aya* must be kept in the casualty area.

Doctors, nurses and paramedical in the emergency area

Emergency area: The moment a patient enters the emergency area, doctors and nurses on duty must immediately attend to the patient, with the doctors diagnosing the problem and the nurses taking vitals. Paramedics should also be on standby as a precautionary measure. If the problem is of RTA or any type of casualty, the paramedic should immediately start assisting the doctor.

Doctors in the casualty area must carry out these duties once they have completed the initial investigation:

1. Provide emergency treatment to the patient and write a prescription.

2. Decide whether the patient should be treated in the day care, ICU, ward or OT after diagnosing the patient's condition; and if necessary, announce code blue. Sometimes, even after giving emergency treatment, doctors advise OPD consultation for them and/or send their specimen(s) for laboratory and diagnostic investigations.

3. Minor OT procedures, stitches, plaster, dressing, etc, should be done in the casualty area.

4. Doctors on duty must decide under whom the patient will be admitted.

5. Prognosis should be explained to the patient's attendant in the presence of the casualty manager.

6. The doctors also shouldn't hesitate to do other miscellaneous work, if required.

Problems an administrative manager may face in a casualty area are:

a. In rare cases, doctors, nurses and paramedics are late in attending a patient for reasons like heavy rush, etc.

b. The on-call consultant does not arrive on time.

c. Important forms are not filled out by concerned staff.

d. Delay in LAMA, referral and shifting.

e. Doctors, nurses and paramedics handing over patient history verbally, failing to maintain the medical records properly. This usually happens during the changeover of staff or due to extremely busy conditions.

An administrator's objective:

1. An administrator must know the importance of shifting patients, so as to keep casualty beds available for the next patients.

2. To provide the best medical care possible to the patients.

Coordination of laboratories & diagnostics department in the emergency area:

The moment a casualty medical officer prescribes a medicine or a test, the nurses on duty should immediately work to promptly deliver the former to the patient or make arrangements to carry out the latter, like sending blood samples for investigation, or informing the relevant department, such as MRI, CT scan, x-ray, ultrasound, etc, about the need to carry out the test.

Sometimes in emergency cases, a patient is directly shifted to the ICU from the casualty ward. The necessary laboratory & diagnostics tests should be carried out in the ICU. To speed up the tests, like electrocardiogram, echocardiogram, x-ray, etc, portable machines are used. Once the patient is stable, then an MRI or a CT scan can be taken.

If a patient is not in need of any further investigation, they should be promptly escorted to the department relevant to their needs.

It is the duty of the casualty manager to ensure all these things occur through efficient supervision and coordination, in order to optimize the care that the patient receives.

Housekeeping in the emergency area:

The housekeeping department should take the utmost care to maintain the strictest standards of hygiene and cleanliness possible in the emergency area.

An administrative manager would face the following issues in the emergency area if the housekeeping staff is not competent or handled properly.

a. Newly appointed housekeeping staff are assigned to work without being properly trained.

b. The housekeeping staff changes frequently, lacking stability.

c. The staff are not using safety items like gloves while clearing waste.

d. The staff focus too much on one patient, leaving others unattended with their vomit, urinate or release stool, which causes those patients great discomfort.

e. Sometimes, male or female housekeeping staff are not available, and as a result, the casualty manager has to call staff from other departments, causing delays and inconvenience for both the patients and the manager.

All these prove how vital the housekeeping department is for a hospital. The recruitment of the housekeeping staff must be carefully done so that only appropriate candidates are chosen. Then, the hospital must train them in the various standard operating procedures.

Rare incident: Generally, it is the duty of the housekeeping staff to bring a dead patient's body to the mortuary. Occasionally, valuables are stolen while the corpse is being transported, which is a serious issue. One such incident occurred when a corpse was hurriedly removed from the casualty area before the patient's attendant could fill a valuables form. The theft was later reported by the dead patient's relatives. It is very difficult to ascertain who is responsible for such thefts, and it is another reason why CCTV systems are important for a hospital.

> *"In the healthcare industry, 'casual attitude' is strictly forbidden. The casualty manager must realize that it is important to fill the valuables form. While handing over the valuables to their relatives, it is imperative that they get the acknowledgement signed to prevent any issue, legal or otherwise, in the future." – VBJ*

Coordination by emergency department – I

[The admission, billing, cashier, and third-party administrator desks.]

In most hospitals, patients are admitted under three categories.

1. Cash category.

2. Panel category.

3. TPA category.

Miscellaneous: A patient who requires only first aid, day care or minor OT procedure or something that doesn't require serious treatment, can pay at the casualty cashier/billing counter and leave, while the patient in the panel category will receive emergency treatment either cashless or pay as per the memorandum of understanding they have signed.

The administrator can face the following problems from the admission, billing, and TPA clearance desks:

a. A road traffic accident (RTA) patient doesn't have money.

b. Unknown patient.

c. A panel patient doesn't have the money or a credit letter to pay admission.

d. LAMA or referral patient.

e. MLC (medico-legal case) patient.

f. A patient who cannot afford to pay the full expenses for their treatment seeking a discount.

g. Private hospitals don't accept cheques, which can cause delay in admissions.

h. A patient who doesn't carry proof of identity.

If any of the situations mentioned above requires the administrative manager to talk to senior management for advice/instructions on how to handle such a patient, he/she must not hesitate to do so.

Coordination of the emergency department – II

[The maintenance, biomedical, and the information technology departments.]

It is the primary responsibility of the maintenance department to ensure that the hospital's infrastructure/ equipment is functioning well, and it is worthy of a state-of-the-art facility. The administrator must coordinate with the maintenance, biomedical, and IT departments to ensure the smooth functioning of emergency services, and that the following equipment are in optimal condition.

1. Electricity/Power.
2. Airconditioning.
3. Telephone.
4. Fan.
5. Fridge.
6. Storage closet/locker/cupboard.
7. Bed.
8. Mattress.
9. Wheel chair.
10. Stretchers.
11. The biomedical department should provide oxygen cylinders, oxygen pipeline, pulse oximeter, monitors, etc, in the casualty area.
12. The IT department should provide computer in casualty area
13. The plumber should ensure the water drainage system is full proof.
14. Other miscellaneous items and appliances.

Some problems a casualty manager faces from the maintenance department:

a. Dysfunctional telephone/intercom system.
b. Malfunctioning computers.

c. Improperly filled oxygen cylinders.

d. Breaking of wheelchairs or stretchers while shifting a patient.

e. Non-functional monitors of casualty area gadgets, like pulse oximeter.

f. Delay in repairing work of various things, like leaking pipes, non-functional appliances, etc.

g. Overflowing drainage system.

h. Unusable or soiled toilets.

i. In rare cases, unavailability of power backup during an electricity outage affects running of electric-run appliances, like airconditioners and geysers.

j. Other miscellaneous issues.

Conclusion:

The maintenance department is the backbone of the hospital, maintaining the necessary infrastructure and essential amenities. They ensure that all the hospital staff can carry out their duties without having to worry about non-functional equipment.

Suggestions:

1. The maintenance department must work around the clock each day of the year to ensure the hospital is functioning well, and do mock drills every 3-4 months to ensure they can cope with emergencies.

2. The maintenance department should take care to regularly inspect all infrastructure and equipment, and have a zero-tolerance policy for improperly done maintenance work.

Coordination of the pharmacy with the emergency area:

The doctors in the emergency/casualty area need easy access to medicine so that they can provide quick and effective treatment to emergency patients. The emergency area generally has all life support medicine, but sometimes a patient needs a more specific type of medicine that has to be purchased from the pharmacy.

The administration manager faces the following problems in coordinating the emergency/casualty area and the pharmacy.

a. In a private hospital, replacing the necessary medicines can result in a delay.

b. The patient does not have the money to pay for the medicine.

c. Sometimes, a doctor will prescribe medicine which is not available in the hospital pharmacy, which means the pharmacist must coordinate with the doctors and the casualty manager to obtain the required medicine from an outside source (or at least locate a suitable substitute) and deliver it to the patient.

The administrator must ensure a swift response from the pharmacy in providing medicine. And if the patient/patient attendants do not have the money to pay, the administrator should also allow a credit facility so that the treatment can continue. After the patient's life has been saved, the administrator can arrange for receipts to ensure that payment is provided later on.

Kitchen services in the emergency department:

In the casualty area, kitchen services are not usually expected. However, when a patient is admitted to the emergency area and has been waiting to be shifted for a long time, the administrator/sister in charge should arrange food and other items for the patient as advised by the consultant/doctor.

An administrative manager would face the following problems concerning kitchen services in the emergency area:

a. There is a delay in food being obtained and delivered to the patient.

b. Patients are given food which is unsuitable for them, such as diabetic patients receiving non-diabetic diet, a patient on a liquid diet being given soft food, a patient on a soft food diet being given normal food, etc.

These can all occur due to miscommunication between the casualty manager/sisters in charge and the kitchen department.

Suggestion: The sister in charge/casualty manager should ensure the kitchen department is aware of a patient's name, number and bed, so that the waiter can know exactly whom to deliver the food.

Storage in the emergency department:

The casualty department has two primary storage areas, both of which should be handled by the nurses and paramedical staff:

1. Medical store

2. Non-medical store.

The nurses and paramedical should also maintain the following things in storage.

1. Crash carts in the casualty area, as per life support protocols for emergencies.

2. Defibrillator: A device used to give shocks to the heart for patients suffering from life threatening cardiac disorders.

3. Electrocardiogram (ECG) machines, blood-pressure measuring instruments, pulse oximeter, oxygen cylinder/pipeline, dressing kits, plasters, catheters, etc.

Some large hospitals have separate stores for back-ups for all these devices, which can be used in emergencies, or shifted from the ICU/ward on short notice.

Reception in an emergency:

The reception is the eyes and ears of the hospital, and the administrator should always keep in touch with the reception staff to ensure:

1. Support and communication facilities.

2. Proper distribution of information across the hospital departments and to the patients concerned.

The receptions should always help and support the casualty staff during urgent situations and disasters such as code blue/code red/code violet incidents. Although modern technology allows for the administrator to have useful devices such as mobile phones and computers at their service to make their job easier, the usefulness of the reception should be not underestimated. Receptions often work around the clock to assist the emergency department in carrying out their duties efficiently.

Coordination of ambulance services by emergency department:

Casualty services are always alert and working around the clock every day of the year to meet every challenge.

1. If a phone call comes requesting for an ambulance, the casualty manager must coordinate with the ambulance services to have one sent to the patient's destination as soon as possible.

2. If a patient wants LAMA/referral, the doctors on duty and the casualty manager can arrange for an ambulance to carry the patient to their hospital of choice.

Apart from the above two points, it has been observed that at night, due to roadside gates being closed in residential sectors, it can take too long for an ambulance to locate the patient and reach their destination. The transport administrator and the night manager can coordinate with the driver to help the latter reach the correct location, as well as avoid other issues such as road diversions or an excess of traffic.

Coordination of MRD department with the emergency area:

Sometimes, patient attendants provide incorrect information regarding the name/age/address of the patient, which can be an issue when creating a death certificate for a brought-dead patient. The administrator should help ensure that the patient attendants provide proper ID proof, Aadhar card and essential documents.

Coordination of laundry department with the emergency area:

The laundry department plays an important role in keeping things such as bedsheets, patient's clothes, curtains, towels, etc, clean, and also ensuring that the emergency area has a sufficient amount of these items in storage.

The sister in charge also looks after non-medical stores pertaining to the laundry department.

If the laundry department is not running properly, administrators face a number of problems wherever requesting bedsheets, blankets, towels, curtains etc, not being able to obtain as many of those objects as required.

Advice: Before giving clothes, like bedsheets or towels, to patients, the ward staff must ensure that they are properly cleaned and don't have dirt or stains on them. If they find such clothes, they must immediately send them back to the laundry department.

Emergency department and coordination with the blood bank:

In the emergency department, the casualty manager rarely coordinates with the blood bank. However, if patient come for a blood transfusion request from another hospital/nursing home/clinic, then the casualty doctors advise admission in day care/ward/ICU depending upon patient's condition. At the same time casualty manager helps in arranging everything from admission to availability of blood, thus, helping the patient in getting best medical treatment.

Emergency department during a disaster:

Emergency services play a very important role in disaster management, with doctors and staff investing all their effort into saving the lives of patients.

A disaster can happen for a number of reasons, like traffic accidents, a fire in the hospital, a bomb blast, an earthquake, a collapsed building, etc. These cannot be predicted, only anticipated as unforeseeable circumstances.

Due to a disaster, many injured people will come to the hospital through ambulances as well as private or public transport, and security officials will have a hard time handling both the crowd and managing traffic movement in this situation.

At a given time, if there are more injured or sick patients coming to the emergency area than normal, then the CMO on duty announces a disaster and establishes a temporary command centre at the medical superintendent's office or some other suitable place, from where the entire operation is coordinated.

The alert doctors and nurses in the emergency area, will place identification tags on each injured patient. For example: black tags for patients who are dead on arrival, red tags for patients in serious condition, yellow tags for moderately injured patients and green tags for first-aid patients.

The members of the core committee responsible for disaster management will arrive with short notice, and then arrange everything from treatment to discharge for patients requiring first aid, ICU/ward/admission procedure. The administrative manager informs the police for MLC formalities or postmortem, as well as maintaining law and order in and around hospital premises wherever required. Disasters cannot be managed without the coordinator's efforts.

The casualty manager helps in shifting black tagged patients to the "brought dead" area if more than one death took place and after that, they will be shifted to the mortuary for further action. This allows the doctors and nurses to put their entire focus on red-, yellow-, and green-tagged patients.

The entire staff should be well versed in handling disasters of any nature and regularly practice mock drills, like the following:

a. Command centre.

b. Safety plan.

c. Assembly plan.

d. Evacuation drill.

e. Other types of mock drills.

These must be done once every three to four months to remain prepared for such incidents.

Conclusions:

a. All the heads of the non-medical departments, such as the chiefs of security, transport, the kitchen, PRO, maintenance, IT, housekeeping, pharmacy, etc, are all vital parts of the disaster management committee along with the medical superintendent/doctors.

b. All the staff in the hospital have specific roles and standard operating procedure (SOP) in discharging their duties. The administrator works as the nerve centre to assist in the successful execution of emergency services without disturbing the hospital's ecosystem.

"The main job of all non-medical staff is to assist doctors in saving the life of a patient, including carrying out all formalities, except treatment – for which medicos are required." – VBJ

Management's role in a casualty department:

The casualty/emergency area is the first line of contact between patients and/or their attendants with the administrator. Often, emotions in an emergency area run high, with patients and patient attendants being mentally clogged by stress, fear of loss – and sometimes hyper aggression. The administrator should always maintain calm and do their best to soothe tensions and arrange the best medical attention possible for patients.

The management always supports the administrator in supervising and implementing standard operating procedures. The administrator should always use their aid to ensure that everything is under control from the entry of patients until their shifting or discharge.

It should also be noted that the administrator is the first person to interact on behalf of management concerning the running of a hospital.

Conclusions:

The administrator should be intelligent, proactive, and resilient in dealing with adversity so as to make sure that the hospital continues to function smoothly.

All the departments of a hospital should work as a team, with the knowledge that even the non-medical staff are crucial in providing the best possible healthcare to the patients.

The emergency department plays a very important role in saving patients coming to the hospital in critical condition. The casualty manager should always be alert while working. Their duties are as follows:

a. To coordinate services and provide urgent medical treatment.

b. To shift the patient as per the doctor's instruction, so that the bed is available for the next patient.

c. To explain the estimated financial expenditure to the patient and/or the patient's attendant during the course of treatment.

d. To explain the prognosis to the patient's attendant in consultation with emergency doctors.

e. To arrange timely MLC for RTA or other suspicious cases, like victims of assault and/or who are brought dead, etc.

f. For patients who arrive dead on arrival: To ensure that important forms are signed, that the dead patient's valuables are handed to their kith and kin, hand over the dead body to the legal heir. If the legal heir is not present, they should be contacted and informed of what has occurred. If the legal heir cannot be convinced, then the police should be informed to avoid any stressful situations later on.

g.   To do their best to identify unknown patients and inform police if identification cannot be obtained.

h.   If calls come for an ambulance, then one should be promptly dispatched to the patient's location.

"Timely intervention, timely action, timely solution is the key attribute of a successful administrator." – VBJ

Lesson 5

Outpatient, preventive check-up and physiotherapy department (OPD)

Once upon a time, doctors used to treat patients at their homes which was considered the only safe place, but with the passage of time, doctors started seeing the patients in private clinics, nursing homes and hospitals. Hence the concept of "outpatient department" started.

The OPD is divided into many specialized facilities within the hospital, and also includes a pharmacy, laboratory, diagnostic, optical shops, cafeteria etc under one roof.

The OPD provides the following facilities:

1. OPD has various specialties depending upon a doctor's qualification and discipline, such as cardiac OPD, dental OPD, surgical OPD, ophthalmology OPD, ear-nose-throat (ENT) OPD, physiotherapy OPD, etc.

2. A helpdesk/registration counter (billing), reception, appointment room, etc.

3. Security guard for maintaining peace and order.

4. Toilet/potable water arrangement.

5. IT, computer section and infrastructure.

6. Non-medical staff for housekeeping, ward boys/*ayas*, nurses, lab technicians, paramedics, dental technicians, receptionists, those handling billing, etc.

7. Immunization room, dietician room and library.

8. Crash cart (life-saving medicine) for patients.

9. Preventive check-up department.

10. An OPD has regular timings, which is normally from 8am to 9pm, but can vary depending upon location/area/local factors.

11. The OPD is open only in a few hospitals on Sundays.

Some common problems an administrative manager faces running the OPD:

a. Sometimes OPD doctors want patients to see a specialist consultant, which causes delays.

b. Sometimes a doctor may leave for a surgery or some other similarly urgent work, which can also cause delays.

c. A doctor sees a patient who jumps the queue or out of turn

d. Sometimes there is no proper arrangement for things a patient might require, such as drinking water, toilet, security guard, and support devices, like wheelchairs.

e. If a doctor comes late, alternate arrangements take a long time.

f. The condition of a patient in a queue area worsens as they wait, and shifting them to the emergency area takes time.

g. Issues with payment, refunds and credit facility for panel patients.

h. Sometimes patients and/or their attendants are anxious and want to see the doctor before others.

i. Sometimes, ward boys/*ayas* bring patients on wheelchairs or stretchers in the OPD and move away leaving them alone. This stresses the OPD manager. In such cases, the OPD manager must be ready with alternative plans to get the patient to see the doctor at the earliest without any problem.

"Handing vulnerable patients with ease is very challenging, but also satisfying if done with empathy. Building trust between the service provider and patients is an absolute must." – VBJ

Role of the administrative manager in the OPD

1. Ensuring implementation of a proper roster for all non-medical staff.

2. To make sure that everyone works as a team and ensure quality patient care.

3. To lead from the front:

   a. To assist and liaison with medical and non-medical staff.

   b. Maintaining machines and materials, like monitors, wheelchairs, bedsheets, emergency crash carts, dressing trolly, oxygen cylinders, etc.

   c. To supervise financial transactions.

   d. Use a public address system for staff/patient information/patient benefit.

   e. Ensure all sign boards/notice boards and the helpdesk are well maintained.

In other words, organizing and synchronization of day-to-day operations in the OPD and supervising daily administrative operation monitoring expenses and suggesting cost effective solutions is the key role of an administrator.

"A key mantra for an OPD manager is: hone skills to handle dissatisfied patients with empathy." – VBJ

Conclusions:

a. The role of the OPD manager is to supervise, guide and monitor the entire OPD operation and ensure it runs smoothly, overseeing things like online appointment, registration, coordination, communication with the patient/attendant, etc. The OPD manager also has access to senior management, in case they need help. The manager should also have zero tolerance for certain things, like theft.

b. To have a clear corridor/passage to other parts of the hospital for an OPD patient whose condition worsens and requires emergency treatment.

c. In case of a fire or other disaster, the manager must oversee the movement of the staff and patients to a safer area.

Therefore, the OPD manager must maintain good coordination with doctors for the patient's benefit to provide the best medical advice possible.

Preventive health check-up department

The preventive health check-up department is part of the outpatient department, which is fully equipped with almost all lab and diagnostic testing facilities.

Each hospital has a preventive healthcare department. It is dedicated to preventing diseases in their early stages before it aggravates.

To provide benefits to the public and working class in the private, multinational, corporate, public sector, and government sectors, a special test is prescribed to look for specific diagnoses. For example, routine heart check-ups will have an echocardiogram (echo), ECG, treadmill test (TMT), etc. Routine checks for diabetics will have blood sugar fasting, haemoglobin A1c (HbA1c) test, microalbumin test, kidney function test, ultrasound test, etc. Routine asthma checks will have x-ray, pulmonary function test, complete blood count test, etc.

Health packages have a 30 to 50 per cent discount rate if the tests are billed separately. The idea is to offer an incentive to the maximum number of people who are healthy and health conscious to come for annual check-ups in the hospital to detect any problems they might have in the early stages so that corrective measures can be taken.

The marketing department also recommends employees from government, public and private sectors for annual check-ups. This includes people selected for joining organizations for employment, where a prior certificate of good health is necessary.

The preventive check-ups start at 8am and continue until 5pm to 6pm, depending upon the workload and infrastructure of the hospital in question.

The preventive check-ups are conducted by doctors, who in turn report to the medical superintendent. The coordinator is a non-medical member or of staff, who takes care of the entire preventive check-up department, handling things, such as billing, testing, refreshments, reports, and consultations with doctors.

The coordinator faces the following common problems:

a.   Some people who have taken medicine for a heart disease come in for a cardiac test. The coordinator should take advice from the doctor and ask them to make a future appointment after discontinuing the some of the medicines they were taking as a part of their ongoing treatment.

[Note: some hospitals allow for preventive check-ups at any time, such as chest x-ray, ECG, etc, on the same day and ask the person to come next morning with an empty stomach for other tests, collect all reports by evening and then help arrange a consultation with the doctor.]

b. People with high blood pressure are generally not allowed to take a treadmill test (TMT).

c. Sometimes oily refreshments are served, which a patient/a person who has come for a test may refuse for various reasons. (In all major hospitals the dietician ensures that refreshments consist of a healthy diet, and whenever any problem arises, the dietician should immediately talk to the person concerned and try to solve the issue at the earliest possible time.)

d. Sometimes a doctor advises patients to consult with another specialty doctor, which the person wants to be shown in the same package. And sometimes, doctors will write more tests which are not included in packages but the patient will insist on the same discount as in the rest of the package they have signed up for.

e. Sometimes, a patient might insist upon taking a Holter test on the same day, even if it is not available.

f. In some rare cases, despite taking all precaution for TMT test, if a person starts complaining about chest pain, heaviness or inability to run, the technician should immediately stop the TMT machine and the on-duty doctor should provide first aid depending upon the condition of the patient. If the condition of the patient worsens and becomes life threatening, announce code blue immediately. The coordinator should arrange safe passage for the person to be shifted to emergency or cardiac ICU for further treatment. The entire staff must be well trained to handle such emergency conditions.

g. Sometimes people want everything quickly, such as a test report and a consultation on the same day or at the earliest for a range of reasons.

h. Generally, office employees come in groups for annual check-ups and expect everything completed for their group on the same day.

i. Other unforeseen problems.

Beware of touts:

Only authorized people who have proper identification should be contacted and/or consulted for any suggestions and/or help. Beware of touts as there are imposters who pretend to be a hospital's representative, but have malicious intentions. They seek to cause harm to the hospital, patients, and staff.

"For any medical check-up report, especially for employment/ promotion/job transfer, the hospital management should strictly follow the guidelines. The reports must be sent in sealed envelopes clearly addressed to the authorized person to receive it, and must be sent through a reliable service, like post or courier. Receipts of the dispatch must be persevered and presented on demand. No information of the reports should be leaked under any condition." – VBJ

Physiotherapy department

The medical superintendent is in charge of the hospital, and the head of the physiotherapist department reports to the medical superintendent for day-to-day issues and takes his/her advice. In most hospitals, the physiotherapy department works in morning and evening shifts. However, in some hospitals, physiotherapists work in night shifts also, generally for ICU patients.

Job profile of physiotherapist:

1. To ensure physiotherapy equipment is functional under annual maintenance contracts.

2. All equipment are well calibrated and are in good working condition.

3. If there is any doubt regarding the treatment of a patient, take advice from consultants/concerned doctors before taking any tasks.

4. To ensure training and continuous medical education for the staff.

5. To carry out timely resolutions to patient problems.

The physiotherapy department faces the following problems:

1. Dysfunctional machines.

2. On off days/holidays, this department is closed in most of the hospitals, although in some hospitals, the department is only closed in the evenings of such days.

3. Sometimes female patients ask for female physiotherapists.

4. In rare cases, due to negligence of on-duty nurses and/or physiotherapists, hot water bottles result in severe burns in drowsy or unconscious patients.

5. In rare cases, patients get mild electric shock through defective equipment.

6. Sometimes patients fall from the bed or while walking or doing exercise during therapy.

7. Other issues.

The chief administrative manager does not interfere in the routine work of the physiotherapy department but whenever an end user is brought to the notice of the admin manager, he resolves the issue with a 360-degree approach.

The motto of physiotherapy: Physiotherapists helps to rehabilitate and restore good health with the help of proper assessment, manual therapy, and exercises.

Challenges faced: Lack of awareness and impatience of patients because physiotherapy treatment takes days of sessions to get relief.

Conclusion: The success of the physiotherapy department depends upon the teamwork of the physiotherapists. A card is issued to monitor the outcome of therapy in every patient. If a patient does not get the benefit on stipulated time, then the head of department should review therapy with the doctor and supervise the case regularly. The non-medicos must check weather all equipment is operational, all processes ranging from billing, to registration, queuing, and coordination of treatment are seamless.

Lesson 6

Intensive care unit (ICU)

Whenever a patient comes to a hospital in a critical state or in a life-threatening emergency, the doctors on duty must immediately provide primary treatment and advise the following:

1. For life-threatening conditions, announce "code blue".

2. For patients in serious condition who do not have stable vitals, doctors are advised to shift them to the ICU.

In both situations, doctors should brief the attendant about the medical condition of the patient in the presence of the causality manager. The causality manager makes all the arrangements to shift the patient to the ICU and to coordinate with the admission/ICU manager for further treatment. Sometimes beds are not available in the ICU, so until one is arranged, the patient must remain in emergency with all life support.

It has been observed that at times, a patient's condition worsens in the ward. The doctors on duty must immediately either announce code blue or make arrangements for shifting the patient to the ICU with the help of staff. On other times, a patient's condition can also worsen during an operation or a procedure. In this case too, the doctor on duty should immediately shift the patient to the ICU to save the patient's life.

The ICU is known by different names according to the specialized treatment required for different patients. For example, the burn ICU, cardiac ICU, medical ICU, trauma ICU, CTVS ICU, neuro ICU, paediatrics ICU, neonatal ICU are all designed for different sorts of injuries and illnesses.

1. **Burn ICU** contains important life-saving monitors, ventilators, crash carts, pulse oximeters, oxygen pipes, dressing trolleys, etc. The non-medical staff, plastic surgeons, doctors and nurses here are well trained in treating burn patients.

2. **Cardiac ICU** contains cardiac monitors, ventilators, temporary pacemakers, intra-aortic balloon pumps (IABP), and other

accessories. Here, cardiologist doctors, nurses and non-medical staff are well versed in handling cardiac emergencies. The catheterization lab/cardiac OT are also located nearby.

The entire team of non-medico staff, such as those for maintenance, laundry staff, housekeeping staff, ward boys, paramedical personnel, nurses, *ayas*, etc, play a crucial role in assisting doctors in treating emergency patients.

Similarly the lab & diagnostic department always works 24/7 to assist doctors in treating patients with life threatening diseases by providing information of lab & diagnostic investigation.

"The role of the ICU is a unique one: to provide life-saving, urgent and ultimate treatment to patients." — VBJ

Role of ICU manager (administrator)

The ICU is one of the most important departments of a hospital. This is the only department where patient relatives and attendants wait outside in the waiting area and are only allowed twice a day in the morning and evening to meet the patient/interact with doctors to learn the current status of the patient. During the entire stay, the patient is closely monitored under the watchful eyes of the doctors, nurses and staff.

The manager of an ICU plays a very important role. They are:

a. To coordinate liaison with doctors, nurses and paramedics, maintenance, billing, laundry, IT, housekeeping staff, etc.

b. To get the prognosis explained by the treating doctor to the patient's attendant and obtaining the attendant's signature on the prognosis form.

c. To coordinate with TPA/panel companies on an SOS basis.

d. To allow panel companies and their doctors (if they come) to arrange meetings with consultants, patients ,and attendants.

e. In case of an MLC case, to coordinate with police officers.

f. To coordinate with the patient's attendant on LAMA or DOR.

g. On doctor's orders help patients to shift to HDU or ward.

h. To help the attendant if a request comes for a second opinion.

i. Help HIC nurses to obtain swab from every part of the ICU for testing.

j. Other miscellaneous duties, like explaining the treatment expenses to the patient's attendant.

Of late, a majority of hospitals have adopted the concept HDU (high-dependency unit) for less serious patients or those patients whose consultants wish for them to be admitted for one or two days for observation. Here, patient care is more or less like the ICU but has the advantage of allowing one attendant to be with the patient on a regular basis, to help boost the patient's morale and confidence. The other protocols are more or less the same as the ICU.

ICU is one of the most work intensive areas in the hospital, and sometimes the patient's attendant fails to accept death in spite of repeated counselling by senior doctors and administrators.

Depending upon the hospital policy, the administrator must work on the following points while treating critically ill patients:

a. On a patient's attendant request, arrange a second opinion by a senior consultant.

b. Provide case summaries of patients with all laboratory & diagnostic reports.

c. If any doctor of an attendant's choice wants to visit the hospital to see the patient, the administrator should brief the medical superintendent and can only allow it if permission is granted. *[Note: Some hospitals don't allow this.]*

d. If a patient's attendant wants to take the patient to their choice of hospital, the administrator should give due respect to their wishes and allow DOR/LAMA.

The administrator should always brief the attendant on everything from treatment to finance in the most dignified and sober language and never react to any provocation. He or she must show empathy and try to resolve any issue amicably.

If the administrator and the on-duty doctor think that in spite of repeated counselling, an attendant is uncooperative and may create problems, the administrator should immediately brief the higher management and the security in charge to take preventive measures to safeguard hospital property and staff.

Advice: Hospital management graduates should be taught about ICU-induced psychosis in detail and the problems that arise in such cases.

Conclusion:

The role of the ICU manager is to coordinate, supervise and assist the ICU department for the benefit of patients. The ICU manager plays the role of bridge between the patients and the hospital and also focuses on solutions for ensuring the smooth running of the ICU department.

Word of caution:

A register is maintained at the ICU gate where details of patients and their attendants are entered. The details include phone numbers of patients and their attendants, addresses, etc. It also records the entry and exit timings of patients in the ICU.

Once, a security guard accessed the personal mobile number of a woman attendant from the ICU gate register and started making obscene calls to her. The woman complained to the hospital authorities. The security department then checked the number from where the calls came and identified it as the mobile number of a security guard in the same hospital. His service was immediately terminated.

The register at the reception and ICU contains personal information of patients and their attendants, like phone numbers. Thus, hospitals have a strict policy of not divulging any personal information to unauthorized people to prevent misuse. If anyone is found guilty of this, strict disciplinary action is taken against the employee.

"Ensure counselling for the patient's attendant in the ICU cabin, where the treating doctor, consultant and administrator are present. Ensure CCTV in the cabin is functional before starting the session. Please don't brief them outside ICU, while standing around ICU, Never talk on mobile while briefing in ICU cabin. Focus on the treatment part only. Never ever react to any provocation by a patient's attendant, be firm and focus on the patient's prognosis. Ensure that the patient's attendant signs on the prognosis report at the counselling cabin. This will be evidence if any dispute arises." – VBJ

Lesson 7

Operation theatre (OT)

The operation theatre is also a very vital department in a hospital. The chief anaesthetist is the head of the operation theatre. The chief anaesthetist is supported by the doctors, OT nurses, OT technicians, ward boy/*aya*, housekeeping staff, security guard, IT staff, etc.

There are two types of operation theatres:

1. **Minor OT:** This is generally available in emergency areas where doctors carry out minor operation procedures by giving local anaesthesia. Here the patient is usually discharged immediately, though in some cases day care is required.

2. **Major OT:** All major operations, like bypass heart surgery, laparoscopic surgery, caesarean delivery (C-section), heart surgery, transurethral resection of the prostate (TURP), orthopaedic surgery, skin grafting, etc, take place.

After the operation, the patients are shifted into the recovery room and then to the ward/ICU/HDU/day care depending upon the condition of the patients.

The operation theatre should be properly sterilized by the hospital infection committee before taking any patient to the operation theatre.

Miscellaneous OTs:

a. Special OT room is provided for bronchoscopy, endoscopy, cataract surgery etc.

b. Catheterization lab also requires anaesthetists and cardiologists to carry out angiography, angioplasty and other cardiac procedures.

Code of conduct for OT:

a. Perform the appropriate procedure on the correct patient.

b. The operation must be done at the correct site.

c. The correct implant must be used.

d. Obtain proper consent, documentation, checklist, and prognosis.

The OT department faces the following administrative problems:

a. Sometimes PAC doctors are not available, thus the operation is delayed for a few hours.

b. Patient is brought for bronchoscopy/ surgery but does not have clearance from the PAC doctors.

c. Patients remain in the recovery room for a long time due to the staff neglecting to arrange their shift to other parts of the hospital.

d. Patients urgently require blood at the eleventh hour of the operation.

e. A patient's condition deteriorates or goes into shock during an operation (though this is rare).

f. A doctor has recommended more tests, thus leading to the operation being delayed because the doctor wants 100 per cent clearance approval before shifting to the operation theatre.

g. The prognosis is not explained to relatives as the patient attendant alleged.

h. Air-handling unit (AHU), AC, maintenance work, etc.

i. An operation might get delayed due to malfunctioning of equipment.

j. Other unforeseen problems.

All above problems, should they arise, may be solved through the collective effort of the medical superintendent, chief anaesthetist and the doctors concerned.

The operation theatre is the only department where a strict protocol for uniforms is followed before going inside. It is a part of strict hygiene and sterility standards. No unauthorized personnel are allowed to enter the OT area/recovery area. Strict protocols are enforced to ensure proper management and disposal of any biomedical waste. The housekeeping department ensures no infection is spread from the blood, tissue or any other body part of the patient. Even hospital infection-control (HIC) nurses coordinate with the housekeeping department and OT staff for systemic disposal of bio medical waste after the operation.

It may sound very strange that the chief administrator has no role in the OT department. The department is purely the responsibility of chief anaesthetist and medical superintendent. However, for some issues involving manpower, storage, IT, laundry, maintenance work, housekeeping, security, etc, the chief administrator coordinates with the OT department and offers help.

Advice: To avoid any unforeseeable issues, the anaesthesiologist must follow hospital guidelines and the checklist for error-free documentation. This includes providing correct information and prognosis to the patient's attendant in writing before taking the patient for surgery. This will help in minimizing any avoidable issue.

Word of caution:

During a live demonstration of a surgery on a patient, the condition of the patient may deteriorate in rare cases. The medical superintendent and the chief anaesthetist must ensure that they avoid showing live demonstrations of delicate/high-risk operations.

"The motto of the OT department is to have absolute success in all procedures, with no errors and absolutely no adverse outcomes."
– VBJ

Lesson 8

Wards

The most habitable place in the entire hospital are the wards. Based on clinical assessments, doctors on duty will decide to shift patients to a ward. One or two attendants are there to help the patients. Some hospitals allow the patient's attendants to come in morning and evening to see their patients. Different arrangements (visitor policy) are enforced depending upon the areas and specialty branches of the hospital.

Problem an administrator faces in wards:

a. The hospital bill estimate and the final amount of money in the actual bill do not match.

b. TPA/empanelment issues.

c. Problems with non-medical support staff, like housekeeping, security, kitchen, maintenance, laundry, laboratories, diagnostics, etc.

d. Problem while shifting a patient, like from ICU to ward or ward to ICU or ward to OT or OT to ward, etc.

e. Coordination issues with doctors, nurses, dieticians, physiotherapists, paramedics, etc.

f. IT problems, like non-functional computers, internet services not working, etc.

g. Code violet, code pink, code blue and code red issues.

h. Patients falling down from the bed or in the toilet.

i. During maintenance of the ward facility while the patient is still in the bed/room, sometimes maintenance workers start repairing TV, fridge, replace tubelights, etc, with no alternative arrangement provided to the patient.

j. Other unforeseen problems.

The ward is the place most vulnerable to conflict, aggression and dissatisfaction. Here the patient is generally conscious and the attendant gets feedback from patients of any dissatisfaction because of medical/non-medical staff. The administrator should immediately focus on solving the problem so that such minor issues can be solved before they fester and require more drastic action by the higher management.

There are four types of patients in wards:

1. **Stable patient:** Admitted to the ward, undergoes treatment and discharged from the ward.

2. **Do-not-resuscitate (DNR) patient:** Here, the patient's attendant knows about the terminal stage of the patient illness.

3. **Unpredictable and uncertain patient (code blue in the ward):** Those patients whose health, vitals, and saturation gets abnormal suddenly here doctors nurses announce code blue to save the patient.

Handling the sudden deterioration of patients is one of the common causes of conflict and aggression. It is very difficult to explain certain things, like sudden fall of blood pressure or pulse going missing or cardiac arrest and death of a patient.

In such cases, the patient's attendant reaction becomes highly unpredictable. If a patient is aged or has been hospitalized for a long time, the chances of conflict between the attendant and the hospital staff are less. However, when such things happen to younger patients, their attendants don't accept death easily. Sometimes, their other relatives and friends gather and create problems.

Therefore, the administrator should brief his/her seniors and the security in charge about the situation so that precautions against any violence and damage to hospital property are taken.

Based on administrator's experience, the following points are generally the cause of conflict:

k. Attendant alleges nurses have given wrong injection or medicine to the patient.

l. On a physiotherapist's advice, a patient is asked to walk and their condition suddenly becomes serious.

m. During dressing by paramedical staff, an artery or vein may rupture causing bleeding and worsening the patient's condition.

n. Doctors have not informed the patient attendants about the prognosis of patients and what all could happen to their patients.

o. Doctors advise for discharge, but suddenly the condition of the patient becomes serious.

p. While eating, drinking food particles or water stuck in the windpipe causes the patient to develop a breathing problem.

q. Sometimes embolism may cause sudden breathlessness and the patient's condition becomes critical.

r. Once a patient dies, financial issues become the focus point. Here the management should listen to their point of view and settle the issue amicably.

Whenever any (rare) death takes place in a ward, the relatives and friends of the dead patient start agitating to know the reason. They always find all types of hospital negligence in this situation. To deal with this, the administrator should coordinate a meeting with all treating doctors and management representatives where grieving relatives are counselled and the cause of the death is explained.

Sometimes, when issues find no amicable solution, even the police can get involved. In such a scenario, police may advise a postmortem examination to know the exact cause of death, despite the cause of death being not an accident.

4. Leave against medical advice (LAMA)/discharge of request (DOR)/referral:

When patients/patients' attendants request a hospital to discharge the patient for any reason, the administrator counsel's them to continue the treatment in the hospital. However, if the patient/attendant still insists, the hospital respects her/his decision. Then the hospital arranges an ambulance to help the patient to reach the hospital of her/his choice.

The problems of medical/non-medical staff are ultimately passed on to the administrator for action. The main job of the ward manager is to solve all the problems pertaining to the patient. The ward manager must be a provider of solutions and make all the arrangements for the smooth running of the wards, such as allocation of staff duties and supervision of all the basics and necessary amenities to patients in wards. They must assist and coordinate medical and non-medical staff to increase the quality of the care the patient receives, including briefing the patient on their medical expenses.

Conclusion:

The administrator must have the confidence in his ability to arrange everything from a patient's entrance to the ward until discharge and work to the patient's satisfaction. That is the ultimate role of the administrator.

Advices:

a. *Ensure the case file has laboratory and diagnostic reports of the same patient before showing it to the consultant. In rare cases, case files contain different patient's reports, which causes embarrassment to the ward manager, nursing in charge, and duty doctor.*

b. *Once a patient is discharged, sometimes it is written on discharge summary that a test report of the patient is to be collected after 3 or 4 days. In such a scenario, the patient must be briefed at the time of discharge to collect the report from the lab and diagnostic department and not from wards.*

c. *A very common problem in ward: When a senior consultant comes for a round, sometimes case files are not available or lab and diagnostic reports are not kept in case files or sometimes patients are not around for a range of things, like gone out for MRI/CT scan or a physiotherapy session, etc. This causes embarrassment to the ward manager/floor coordinator, nursing in charge and the duty doctor.*

Root-cause analysis: In most cases, a ward manager/floor coordinator sends a case file to the TPA department for the current status of the patient or the billing department to know the latest expenditure incurred or a radiologist may want to see the case file before any procedure. The ward manager or the administrator must ensure the availability of all lab and diagnostic reports before a senior consultant's visit to the ward. The ward manager or the administrator must ensure that the patient's case file is sent to TPA or billing once the consultant has seen the case file of the patient.

*[**Note:** Based on economic status of patients, a hospital has different categories of wards, like general, semi-private, single-private, single-deluxe, super-deluxe wards and suits. Also, based on specialty of*

treatment, a hospital has different arrangements, like pediatric wards for children, gynae ward for women, etc.]

"The ward manager has to strike a balance between consultation, treatment and reporting for the type of admitted patients such as general cash-based admissions, third party admissions via insurance, and panel companies like CGHS, so that the patient doesn't suffer."
– VBJ

Lesson 9

Nursing department

The most disciplined and well-documented department of a hospital is the nursing department. Love, care, and compassion – all of these are qualities required of nurses. This department is the backbone of the hospital's services. The nursing department is run by a "nursing rule book". All protocols, checklists, etc, are mentioned in the nursing manuals. In order to become a nurse, one must go through extensive training and apply to the nursing council of registration, and then they can join the nursing department. There are also many books on nursing available written by scholars and teachers. Even the National Accreditation Board for Hospitals and Healthcare Providers (NABH) and National Accreditation Board for Testing and Calibration Laboratories (NABL) manuals on nurses are upgraded and taught by nursing tutors and quality managers to improve the care that patients receive.

The nursing department is headed by the nursing superintendent. The nursing superintendent directly coordinates with the MS/administrator/ HR department on an SOS (emergency) basis with management in case of any problems. Nurses in charge on duty manage round-the-clock all kinds of nursing services, such as working to provide better care to the patients by any means by using their vast experience to their advantage. When there is a large number of patients, the nurses in charge fill gaps by:

a. By assigning double duty to nurses by calling them from their hostel or residence.

b. Rotate 8 to 12 hours' duty to ensure nurses can cover all the work in the hospital.

The motto of the nursing department is **zero tolerance for error**. By and large, nurses carefully follow checklists and the doctors' orders. Despite this, there are two types of errors which may occur:

a. Manageable errors.

b. Non-manageable errors.

Manageable errors:

Manageable errors are the following types:

a. Medicine was not given to the patient on time.

b. Blood samples were not collected in time.

c. Blood samples took more than one prick with the needle to obtain.

d. Patient IV/cannula/central line issue/blood oozes out from cannula during the night.

e. The bed-ridden patient gets bed sores.

f. Wrong indentation of medicine.

g. Referrals are not provided to consultants and failure to follow the doctor's orders.

h. Language problems.

i. Unseen fungus in fluids (IV bottle), in rare cases. *[**Note:** The nurse must check if the fluid is transparent and free from any foreign body before using it on a patient. She should also check the expiry date of the IV fluid/medicine.]*

j. Syringes used to feed patients are washed in the bathroom.

k. In rare cases, a patient's file shows that the patient was administered a complete course of medicines/injections for a certain number of days. However, physical stock shows a mismatch.

j. Other miscellaneous issues.

As long as the patient is getting relief and is alive, these are manageable errors. Once the fault is found and brought to the notice of the nursing superintendent, she handles the staff as per the seriousness of the case and the administrative manager also sometimes knows the issue. The nursing superintendent handles the issue with all due sensitivity and tries to settle the problem with a progressive and holistic approach.

Non-manageable errors:

Non-manageable errors are the rarest of rare types of sentinel events or medical errors. They often result in serious conditions for the patient. Some of them are:

a. Wrong site surgery

b. Foreign body retention

c. Other unforeseen serious error

The non-manageable issues are those where gross negligence is reported. The nursing superintendent must sort out the issue with the help of the CEO/MS/management representative or administrator.

Every hospital has an ethical committee to look into the cause of negligence/serious error or death. The chief administrator is also part of the committee.

Note: Manageable and non-manageable issues mentioned are based on practical experience of the author.

Mistakes, large or small, from any employee are not accepted by hospital management and all efforts are made that no life is lost due to negligence. The nursing tutor and quality manager constantly teach and upgrade nurses' knowledge in order to achieve zero error and improve the nurses' management of a patient's care.

Administrative problems nursing services face in the house

The administrative issues hospital nursing services commonly face:

a. Too much workload on the nurses at times. It has been observed that sometimes the nurse-to-patient ratio is 1:10 or even more. This becomes a big issue when the nurses are expected to manage the patients to complete their routine work, going to different consultants to follow their instructions and to take rounds.

b. Sometimes, the number of nurses quitting the hospital for better career prospects exceeds the management's expectations. This causes problems.

c. These days, an increasing number of nurses ask for their rights, like better working hours and conditions. As a result, the nursing superintendent's job is a little tougher than before.

The administrator should always coordinate with the nursing superintendent to sort out administrative issues, if any, in the best interest of the hospital.

"Mistakes, big or small, by anyone aren't accepted by hospital management. All effort must be made that no life is lost due to negligence, precision of approach, etc, with no room for error." – VBJ

Lesson 10

Laboratories & diagnostics department

The laboratories & diagnostics department is the most trusted and reliable department in the hospital. All doctors depend upon the laboratory & diagnostics reports of the patients to identify the illness correctly and plan the best-possible treatment in OPD/IPD/ICU. A patient's admission, medicines, operation, and discharge procedures depend upon the reports received from the laboratories & diagnostics department.

The laboratories & diagnostic department is headed by the MD pathologist and MD radiologist respectively. The laboratories & diagnostic services run around the clock to provide reports to doctors and patients.

For smooth running of the department, non-medicos are appointed as coordinators. Their main job is to coordinate with OPD, walk-in patients and IPD patients.

Problems the laboratories & diagnostic coordinator commonly faces:

a. Delay in getting reports because of slow processes.

b. Unavailability of doctors on Sunday evenings in most of the hospitals. (They are available on call.)

c. In rare cases, incorrect reports can become a serious issue.

d. Sometimes, female patients insist for female radiologist for ultrasound or procedures. The unavailability of a female radiologist during those particular times may cause delay.

e. Security issues (bag, mobile, etc, stolen from the premises).

f. Delay in MRI/CT scan/ultrasound and other procedures.

g. Outsourcing problem, if any.

h. Diagnostics films go missing during shifting a patient from one place to another. In such a scenario, the administration manager asks for a duplicate film to meet statutory requirements of TPA/panel/hospital.

i. Sometimes, patients' condition may worsen during treatment, like sudden drop in blood platelets in dengue patients. In such cases, the treating consultant should explain the patient and/or their attendant and advise them. The administrator/manager/coordinator job is to arrange a meeting between the patient's side and the treating doctor at the earliest.

j. Sometimes, patients insist to crosscheck their laboratories & diagnostics reports with other centres, but most of the hospitals don't allow this. This may cause some resentment on the patients' side. In such cases, the administrator should step in and make the patients' side understand the hospital's policy.

The floor manager ICU Manager/ OPD Manager always coordinates with the laboratories & diagnostics department to help and get reports in time. All doctors and staff are interested in enhancing their profile, hence from time to time, they upgrade their knowledge with continuous medical education. The administration manager does not get involved in day-to-day operations on the clinical side. However, if any end user complains, then the administration manager resolves the issue by arranging meetings with the pathologist/radiologist on the SOS basis of the patient so that the patient's confidence in the hospital is not shaken.

The laboratories & diagnostic department follows the strict guidelines and policies laid down by the Atomic Energy Regulatory Board (AERB) and the Pre-Natal Diagnostic Techniques (PNDT) Act, 1996. Strict protocols are followed for the management and disposal of biomedical waste

The laboratories & diagnostic department also has hospital infection control (HIC) nurses who take swab samples from wards/ICU/OT and other areas to inform the medical superintendent or pathologists or the concerned department about infections, if any, to take corrective and/or preventive actions.

Word of caution:

Sometimes, staff's casual approach on Sundays or holidays can result in embarrassment for the hospital. Let us have a look at such a case and analyse it.

Case study:

Once, on Holi festival, a doctor recommended neck angiography and blood test for a patient at 8am. The sister in charge sent the blood sample to the laboratory while keeping the patient on an empty stomach. After keeping the patient without food for six hours at 2pm, she shifted the patient to the CT department for the procedure. As it was a holiday, the CT department was open until 1.30pm. *[Note: On such days, the CT department opens only on SOS calls after it closes earlier.]*

After keeping the patient waiting outside the CT department for 30 minutes, the patient's attendant was told to come after two hours. This irked the patient's attendant and he got very angry. The administrator had to intervene and apologize to the patient and his attendant on the hospital's behalf. He assured them that the procedure would be carried out on that day itself, but a while later due to unavoidable circumstances. The attendant then decided to bring the patient the next day as the patient was a diabetic and was very hungry being on an empty stomach for so long. Apart from this, the patient was not in a serious condition.

This solved the problem. However, this also exposes the lack of coordination between diagnostics managers and ward managers.

Root-cause analyses:

1. The laboratory & diagnostics department had sent a circular on account of Holi festival the MRI and CT department will function only until 1.30pm and would be opened only during an emergency. However, the laboratory & diagnostics manager just put the circular on the notice board and didn't send it to the dispatch section to be informed of the early closure of the department to concerned departments.

2. If the ward manager had informed the CT department that a patient would come for neck angiography at 2pm, the technician would have waited until that time.

Advices:

a. *The staff should work with full focus while on duty. It doesn't matter whether it is an off day or a holiday. This would avoid situations as mentioned above and cause harassment to patients and embarrassment to the hospital.*

b.   The laboratory & diagnostics department staff should always respect the privacy of patients and never reveal their diseases and other reports to unauthorized people, including the patients themselves. This is the job of the consulting doctor.

"The goal of the laboratories & diagnostic department is to deliver patient reports timely with zero error. This is the key to customer loyalty." - VBJ

Lesson 11

Blood bank department

All major hospitals have a blood bank department. It is either run by the hospital itself or is outsourced. The head of the blood bank reports to the medical superintendent. Non-medical professionals work in the blood bank as coordinators and counsellors, who aid in filling out forms, donor cards, billing, etc.

The blood bank coordinator faces the following issues:

1. Sometimes donors are not available.

2. Sometimes donors are available but do not have the same blood group as the patient.

3. a. In north India, the dengue season mainly starts in August and ends in November. This is a time when many patients require platelet supplements, which increases the demand for platelets many times more than in other months. b. During the Covid-19 pandemic, a huge surge in demand for plasma was observed.

4. Some RTA cases require urgent blood components.

5. Senior citizens requiring blood transfusions don't get any help from their friends and relatives.

6. Generally, migrants who require blood don't have their relatives and friends in the same area and find difficulties in arranging for blood for transfusions.

7. Sometimes TPA insurance never approves the whole amount mentioned in the bill.

8. Other miscellaneous issues.

If any problem occurs, the non-medical administrator always looks at it from every point. However, whenever the administrator of the blood bank isn't able to solve problems, he/she takes the help of the medical superintendent/chief administrator to sort out the issue quickly.

Observation: Generally, people don't come forward to donate blood on their own. To encourage people to do so, the blood bank department keeps on arranging general awareness events, blood donation camps, public lectures, painting competitions, etc, to boost the confidence of the general public from time to time.

The marketing and administration department guides the blood bank in getting permission to arrange blood donation camps, auditoriums for public lectures, etc. They also send invitations to the media for publicity.

The motto of the blood bank department is *"create awareness to donate blood to save lives"*.

Challenge for hospital planners: In India, the number of blood banks are inadequate based on the population, which is an administrative challenge. Inhouse blood banks do not exist in small hospitals, thus the pressure falls on big hospitals to meet demands of those requirements, and external requests from nursing homes and smaller hospitals.

Advice: The administrator must not allow unethical practices in and around blood banks. The department must keep touts away. Sometimes drug addicts come to donate blood for money. Keep an eye on them and report to the security department if any such person comes to notice.

Lesson 12

Central sterile supply department

The central sterile supply department (CSSD) is a very important department that ensures sterilization of all instruments used by medicos, nurses, paramedics, and technicians. Non-medicos having diplomas in CSSD, staff who have an OT technician diploma or experienced people join the CSSD department.

As many high-tech instruments and materials used for medical and surgical intervention are very expensive, most of them are designed in such a way that they can be re-used with 100 per cent sterilization.

The CSSD functions are as follows:

1. Receive contaminated goods.

2. Clean the contaminated goods using standard protocols.

3. Assemble the disassembled goods using standard protocols.

4. Sterile the goods using standard protocols.

5. Store the goods using standard protocols.

6. Supply the goods to the various departments as required.

7. Disposal of waste and infected items. *[**Note:** They are first drained into a tank where a disinfection protocol is well placed. Then those items are sent to a municipal drain.]*

There is no shortcut when it comes to quality. A CSSD technician checks all the disinfected items before they are supplied. Even if a minute error is detected by check indicators, technicians recall all the goods and re-start sterilization until they have 100 per cent infection-free items. The laundry, housekeeping and laboratories staff directly and indirectly coordinate with CSSD for better results. The administration manager does not interfere in the day-to-day operation of CSSD. However, whenever any issue is brought to the notice of the administration manager he or she immediately works to resolve the issue.

Common problems CSSD technicians face:

a. Machine breakdowns.

b. Personal protection suits, hazardous material suits and specialised protection gear such as gloves and goggles are not available.

c. Inadequate chemical indicators used in machines.

d. Unclean or unhygienic stores.

e. Inadequate fire-safety and/or pest-controls in stores.

The CSSD is also supervised by HIC nurses and technicians to randomly check any defect in the supply-chain system and working methodologies of the machine.

The CSSD also runs around the clock every day of the year in most major hospitals. Usually, a pathologist is responsible for the CSSD. The CSSD always keeps stocks of sterilized equipment in store and whenever any demand comes from any department and delivers immediately so that the patient does not suffer.

Conclusion: The CSSD is the lifeline of the hospital, which assists all doctors, nurses and technicians to perform without any fear of infection by providing 100 per cent sterilized linen, instruments, PVC items, etc, for use.

Thoughts for policymakers:

The CSSD is a large and important department. Due to the latest technology and advancement of science, the importance of the CSSD increased greatly. The success of the hospital depends upon an infection-free environment during procedures or operations. Thus the CSSD has become the benchmark for the success of hospital services. It is a specialized department and still untapped for hospital administration graduates at the senior level.

Academic institutions should include specialized subject of CSSD in their syllabus in details, like:

a. Different types of sterilization.

b. Types of autoclave.

c. How autoclaving kills microorganisms.

d. Hospital infection control.

e. Checklist or standard operative procedure for each CSSD function, rather than including just one chapter of CSSD in their courses.

A fully infection-free environment and sterilization in hospitals benefits three classes of people in a hospital – doctors, non-medical class/support staff, and patients.

There are still many opportunities for growth and very promising career options that have not been tapped by hospital administrator graduates.

Conclusion: The CSSD provides full cover from infections to doctors, nurses and technicians from contaminated instruments so that they can carry out their duties confidently.

Lesson 13

Admission and billing department

The admission desk, billing counter, billing counsellor, billing cashier are some non-medical occupations in the healthcare industry. A billing in charge or a billing manager heads the admission and billing department.

Admission desk

Whenever any doctor recommends patients for admission, either in day care, ward or ICU. The patient or its attendant goes to the admission counter for the same.

The admission clerk gets all the relevant demographic details, like name, father's name, address, age, mobile number, gender, TPA panel, cash panel, etc. For unconscious patients and/or unknown patients, the admission clerk makes a file and at the same time informs the MS/administration manager/casualty manager regarding the unknown patients and updates the patients' credentials as and when he or she gets information from authentic sources.

The admission clerk is always in touch with the billing counsellor by providing patients estimates or in case of serious patient CGHS/ECHS beneficiary coordinating in getting an emergency certificate, which is a must for government patients.

Some common problems an admission clerk faces are as follows:

a. A patient attendant writes the wrong name, incorrect address, age, gender, etc, in the form.

b. Patients want cancellation of TPA and to get another TPA for treatment purposes.

c. Some patients do not carry money in an emergency.

d. Some patients want to change doctors in OPD/IPD specialty.

e.   Other miscellaneous problems.

An admission desk should be polite and courteous in dealing with patients. The admission desk requires ID proof and order by the billing manager to carry out any correction in the admission file. Sometimes in RTA/assault cases an attendant wants an MLC after three or four days of admission. Here again the admission clerk should bring this to the notice of a higher authority for correction(s), if any.

Billing desk

The billing desk handles multiple tasks. In the OPD area, the billing clerk does registration as well as collection of cash. In the IPD department, the billing clerk prepares the bill amount for the patient and the cashier collects the payment and hands over all the patient's discharge papers.

Some hospitals have billing counsellors. They are appointed mostly for the following four reasons:

1.   To provide a day-wise estimate.

2.   To provide an estimate before any procedure, like angiography, endoscopy, colonoscopy, OT procedure, etc.

3.   To provide estimates to the TPA/corporate claims panel.

4.   Advise to collect the payments from patients if the bill exceeds the package amount. Such cases happen when the actual amount exceeds the sanctioned amount in packages.

Some of the common problems a billing in charge or a billing counsellor faces are the following:

a.   Sometimes the number of days is wrongly mentioned in a bill.

b.   Sometimes blood samples are taken twice by mistake and billed, angering the patient. The administration manager/MS helps reach an amicable solution.

c.   Sometimes oxygen is not given to patients but is mentioned in the bill.

d. MLCs are not mentioned in the file but charged MLC billing.

e.   Doctors/procedures/OT wrongly charged.

f.   Sometimes there are errors in the billing of dialysis/ bronchoscopy/ procedures, etc.

g.   Physiotherapy charges twice as mentioned but patients get once in a day.

h.   X-ray missing but charged in a bill. As a result, duplicate x-ray films provided by the billing in charge to satisfy patients. It is also a statutory requirement in TPA/panel company cases.

i.   Ripple bed charges are mentioned but were not provided to the patient.

j.   Sometimes blood samples are not taken but charged in the file.

k.   Sometimes urine samples remain in the ward but are charged in the file without culture reporting.

l.   Sometimes ICU charges are shown one day more in a patient's bill, but the patient stays in the ward on the same day.

m.   Sometimes corporate and panel discounts are not mentioned.

n.   The patients' attendant does not show an ESI/CGHS/ECHS card at the time of admission but shows at the time of discharge, resulting in unnecessary delays to modify the bill.

When a panel/TPA patient gets discharged, medicine is not returned, and a bill is made. When it is brought to the notice of billing in charge, the medicine is returned, and the bill is modified and settled.

Advice: The billing in charge must crosscheck the return of medicines from wards and ICUs for TPA/panel companies before making the final bill as it has been observed that sometimes sisters in charge or ward managers unwittingly forget to return the unused medicines. This would avoid unnecessary stress for the billing in charge and the pharmacy later on.

Case study:

Once, a bill was attested by the billing department with the billing manager signing it without checking the government forms properly. The bill was sent to the government for reimbursement, but it was returned without clearance to the patient with a query. When this bill was brought to the notice of billing in charge, the billing in charge found that the date of admission and the date of discharge were wrongly entered in the government form.

*[**Note:** A billing manager should attest any such claim form only after thoroughly going through it and tallying the information with the records. This will cut down incidences like the above and avoid unnecessary trouble for both the patient and the hospital.]*

Billing is an around-the-clock work. There are two or three shifts in the hospital for the billing department depending upon the hospital's policy. For example, the OPD generally works in morning and evening shifts but in case of IPD, the hospital has a maximum of three shifts for billing staff.

Billing managers play a very important role in the corporate claims panel/TPA/government/public sectors/private sector. In corporate claims, bills are processed and sent to the hospital's marketing department for recovery and for payment.

*ced **Advice:** The billing in charge must prepare all bills as per the established protocol or according to the memorandum of understanding with companies to avoid monetary loss.*

Thought for policymakers:

Graduates from hospital administration should be encouraged to join the billing department at a senior level. Academic Institutions should include maximum material in the course curriculum in these fields. It is a very specialized field for non-medicos still untapped by hospital administration graduates. As a result, other candidates are taking these jobs instead. If given proper exposure/training and education of billing as a specialized subject, a hospital administration graduate will do much better than others in this field and take the hospital to the next level of billing, thus creating more job opportunities for career growth.

Above all, the mood of the promoter/owner of a hospital depends upon the following:

1. Correct billing.
2. Smaller crowds in the billing department.
3. No deduction on TPA/panel billing.
4. No delay in preparation of bills.

The above points result in error-free billing.

"The billing department should keep in mind all protocols and MoUs before passing any bill for reimbursement." – VBJ

Lesson 14

Third-party administration (TPA) department

[Processing insurance claims.]

All private and semi-private hospitals have patients who are covered by insurance. They are mostly from public sectors, private sectors, and multinational companies. There are also many patients who are covered by individual insurance (TPA panel). Therefore, the TPA department is a very important department for every hospital. The hospital management graduates are joining the marketing department to look after the TPA business, which is a very challenging job. Some of the hospital graduates also join as TPA manager/TPA coordinator to deal with TPA companies and their main job profile is to coordinate with TPA companies to get approval for patients' treatment expenses.

TPAs are divided into two types:

1. Government associates, like Oriental Insurance Company (billing as per General Insurance Public Sector Association or GIPSA rate).

2. Private insurance companies, like FHPL, Max Bupa, etc, which approve hospital rates (or as per MOU signed with them).

*[**Note:** In the near future, all hospitals may follow rates fixed by General Insurance Public Sector Association (GIPSA).]*

The hospital authorizes doctors to make pre-authorization/reply against queries and discharges. The working in the TPA generally starts from 8am to 9pm in most of the hospitals to get insurance claims cleared. In most of the hospitals, there is no night shift for this department. However, in certain cases of death or emergency, the TPA desk sends for approval and discharges at night for early clearance. Normally it takes two to three hours to get approval from an insurance company.

Job profile of a TPA manager:

a. To send pre-authorization of patients, sending running bills from time to time, and sending case summaries prepared by doctors to update the insurance company regarding the patient's condition.

b. To brief patient attendants about feedback queries raised by insurance companies.

c. Coordinate with doctors and staff on matters pertaining to insurance coverage.

d. Any abnormal behaviour of the attendant is to be reported immediately to the security in charge and the admin manager.

e. Other miscellaneous issues.

Some of the common problems a TPA manager faces are:

a. Co-payment issues, adjustments with amount deposited.

b. Various issues concerning the patient's bill. Examples: i. When a patient is admitted for surgery, but doctors postpone surgery due to unavoidable reasons. ii. Sometimes, TPA executives deny cashless facility to the patient claiming that the patient was admitted for diagnostic/investigation purpose, under which cashless facility is unavailable.

c. Non-payment issue.

d. Surgeon's fees approved by assistant surgeon's fees denied.

e. No confirmation from TPA in spite of frequent reminders.

f. Documentation is not handed over as per TPA requirements.

g. TPA and MOU do not permit gallbladder surgery, bypass surgery or major surgery.

h. Sometimes the final bill amount sent to TPA is more than the package amount.

i. Estimates of ortho surgery are given but the final amount exceeds the estimated amount.

j. Sometimes patients have TPA but no claim number, for which the TPA executive mails to a higher authority to sort out the problem. It generally happens concerning corporate health insurance holders.

Observation: It has been observed that when the TPA sends letters denying treatment for patients, the patient's attendant thinks that it is the hospital's fault. Sometimes lack of coordination and miscommunication results in hot arguments where seniors have to intervene to sort out by taking a progressive and holistic approach.

Advice: Early detection of the problem will give hospital managers an opportunity to sort out the issue at the earliest to avoid untoward incidents.

Conclusion: The TPA is a very sensitive department, like the billing department. Lots of problems present themselves every day on a routine basis. Some of them are:

a. Cashless denial.

b. Death cases.

c. MLC cases.

d. Differential amount to be paid (room difference, proportional charges deduction, etc).

e. Sometimes, consumables are not paid by TPA.

f. Co-payment issue.

g. Other unforeseen problems

The TPA manager should never react to any provocation by patients or patients' attendants personally or over phone or e-mail. In such cases, the administration manager must be involved to sort out the bill issue.

Thoughts for policymakers:

It has been observed that certain cases regarding TPA cause friction between the patients and hospitals. For example, patients with mental/psychiatric problems, dental problems, HIV, or RTA patients who were driving under the influence of alcohol are denied TPA coverage. However, the hospitals cannot deny treatment to such patients just because they are not covered by TPA. Policymakers for TPAs must address such issues and make it clear to the insurance policy holders at the time of issuing policies to them that the cost of treatment won't be covered under the insurance policy in such cases.

If there are amendments in policies regarding such cases, hospitals must be immediately informed.

This will reduce a major cause of friction between the patients and the hospitals.

"The key to resolve TPA issues expeditiously is to have early communication with the patient/attendant as well as the insurance company to avoid miscommunication and glitches." – VBJ

Lesson 15

Accounts, finance, secretarial and legal departments

The accounts, finance, secretarial and legal departments are crucial to the running of the hospital. They are staffed with non-medicos. In most major hospitals, the CMD, managing director or the owner of the hospital directly supervises these departments. They work under senior officials (non-medicos) and have their own working module, but follow the HR guidelines for basic amenities like uniforms, working hours, salary perks, leaves, holidays, etc.

The administrator of the hospital doesn't interfere in day to day activities of all the above mentioned departments but whenever any problems pertaining to the above arises, the administrator talks to the person concerned and sorts out the problem.

Accounts and finance departments

The accounts and finance departments handle and keep records of all financial transactions in the hospital, including salaries and wages of all staff, both medicos and non-medicos.

The most common problem concerning these departments in all hospitals are:

1. **Cash payment:** In spite of modernization, technological advancements, and digitalization, cash transactions are still a mode of payment in all major hospitals. Of late, money-transaction apps (like UPI, Paytm, Google Pay), credit cards and debit cards are gaining popularity. However, a major problem is that when a patient or his/her attendant has to pay an amount of more than ₹2 lakh even when the bill crosses that amount. This is because government regulations don't allow hospitals cash receipts of more than ₹2 lakh. Many people find it difficult to pay through cards for various reasons, like they don't have enough in their bank accounts to pay through debit cards

or not enough credit balance in their credit cards. Also, many raise money for paying medical bills by borrowing or getting the sum through donations, which are mostly in cash. Therefore, cash payments are a serious issue in most hospitals.

2. Very few hospitals accept foreign currency.

3. Many hospitals have the policy to refund any sum above ₹10,000 by transferring the amount directly to the patient's or his/her attendant's bank account. However, at times, the patient or his/her attendant may insist on cash refund for a range of reasons. Such scenarios become very stressful for the administrative manager. During such situations, the administrative manager must try to convince the patient or his/her attendant to accept the hospital's policy. However, the administrative manager may coordinate with the accounts department to make a cash refund in rare cases.

4. Most hospitals don't accept cheques for fear of getting bounced, which is also a big problem. The administrator is always seen coordinating and counselling with the mode of payment.

5. Sometimes, online bank transfers, like NEFT and RTGS, don't show up in the system or the bank's records instantly. However, the patient or his/her attendant insists that the payment has been made and their money has been debited from their account. Such a situation becomes very problematic for the administrative manager as both the hospital and the patient's side believe they are right. Waiting till the account department gives clearance by confirming from the bank causes stress. This also results in unnecessary occupation of beds just for clearance from account departments.

[Note: Discharged patients occupy beds for want of clearance from the billing department and sometimes the payment deposited by an attendant arrives after 3 or 4 hours, which is always a problem in all hospitals. The administrator is always seen busy in coordinating with the concerned departments in minimizing the time gap and always works towards speedy clearance of the bills to get beds vacant for the next patient.]

Suggestion: Payment is always one of thorniest issues in all private hospitals. Hospital management graduates must be taught how to handle payment issues in IPD patients. Sometimes, a discount is given to buy peace or sometimes the balance amount is waived off by showing a discount. In many hospitals, as a thumb rule, 80 per cent of the total estimated bill must be deposited before a treatment, surgery or procedure. Sometimes, even TPA doesn't approve some non-consumable items and/or 3H tests. As a result, hospitals take ₹5,000 to ₹10,000 as advance deposit from them. This sometimes leads to a conflict between the patient or his/her attendant and the hospital. For corporate TPA, many hospitals don't take any advance from patients or their attendants to maintain their business ties.

Future mode of payments in a new era:

In the future, popular cryptocurrencies, like bitcoin, may be accepted in India for business transactions in addition to the existing modes of payment. For this, the existing tax-deduction mechanism will have to be remodelled and upgraded in the hospital's accounts and finance department. Therefore, more non-medicos staff with requisite IT skills will be hired to handle the hospital's account and finance departments.

"In the future, current modes of payments will be rendered redundant. Therefore, it is imperative that the present-day administrative manager must be trained to handle future modes of money transactions." – VBJ

Secretarial and legal department

A smooth-functioning secretarial department is very important. This is because most private hospitals have a corporate setup, which are run as private limited companies. Therefore, they have to comply with laws governing companies. One of the mandatory requirements is to appoint a qualified company secretary (non-medico), who is the first officer in the eyes of the law and answerable to the board of directors for corporate governance. He/she is also responsible for ensuring legal compliance, publishing true and fair accounts as well as taking into account all liabilities to avoid any future non-compliance issue.

The administrator doesn't have a direct link to the secretarial department, but still needs to have a close official relationship to get legal guidance if documentary support is required as evidence in a legal issue. To this end, hospital management graduates must also be taught medical laws, medical negligence, MLC, etc, and how to avoid medical negligence in hospitals by remaining active, alert, agile in implementing and documenting compliance with standard operating procedure and checklists without any fail.

In essence, a secretarial department is a back office meant for taking care of the perpetual issues concerning finance, income, expenditure, and concerns regarding corporate governance. The administrator facilitates all this by ensuring implementation, compliance, and adherence.

Thoughts for policymakers:

New trends and emerging issues pose new challenges in the healthcare sector. To tackle them, hospitals need to do the following:

a. Be prepared to resolve complaints lodged by aggrieved patients or their kin.

b. Medicolegal remedies need to be taught in hospital management courses so that future administrators can handle complaints judiciously.

c. Hospitals should have a legal cell to handle all those complaints which go to courts.

"Importance of the legal department in hospitals will increase manyfold with a sharp rise in the demand for lawyers specializing in cases related to the healthcare sector." – VBJ

Lesson 16

Store and pharmacy

Non-medicos are responsible for running the store. There are different types of stores in hospitals. It depends upon the nature of goods and products stored. For example:

a. Pharmacy stores with medicine, drugs injection, ophthalmic, surgical items, etc.

b. Maintenance store keeps hardware, electrical computers, electronics, etc.

c. Catheterization laboratory store keeps stents and catheterization laboratory items.

d. Central store, where hospital stationaries are warehoused.

The rationale of having a store department in hospitals is to keep an inventory of goods, medicine, etc; and replenish them whenever required. The store in charge does take total supervision of the day-to-day consumption of goods and places orders as and when required. Store managers should keep a regular account of the stock of materials in and out. Stored items are to be utilized on a "first come, first out" (FIFO) basis.

Common problems store managers face:

a. Shortage of goods.

b. Defective goods received.

c. Expired goods or near-expiry goods are not being removed.

d. High inventory of non-moving and slow items and no proper utilization plan.

e. Coordination problems with the purchase department.

f. Other miscellaneous issues.

The administrative manager is generally not involved in the day-to-day operation of the store. However, if the store manager/end user apprises the administrative manager of a problem that the former is unable to handle, the latter tries to understand the real issue with the head of the store and tries to resolve the issue.

Periodically, the head of the store meets the CEO/MS/administrative manager to sort out store-related issues, like maintenance, lack of storage space, storage of medicines and equipment, and also other miscellaneous issues.

The only store which has a retail outlet in a hospital is a pharmacy store. The pharmacy has two outlets:

a. IPD outlet or in-house patients consumption of medicine, implant, stents, cannula, IV sets, CPR kit, etc. This outlet also delivers medicine for TPA, panel companies and cash patients admitted.

b. Retail pharmacy: This outlet caters to OPD patients, walk-in patients from other hospitals with doctors' prescription. Patients getting discharged get their medicine from this outlet. Medicine prescribed by doctors for the casualty department is also sold from here.

The head of the department of the pharmacy is an experienced professional having a bachelor's or master's degree in pharmacy. Of late, online pharmacy networking has gained momentum in some major hospitals and a new concept of "delivering medicine to your doorstep" has emerged.

Common problems a pharmacy manager faces are:

a. Managing cash counters as multiple customers visit at the same time and want to get medicine quickly.

b. Once medicine is sold, it is not returned very easily.

c. Medicine from cold chains cannot be replaced once sold.

d. Products nearing their expiry dates remain sold.

e. Medicines prescribed by the consultant are unavailable.

f. Wrong medicine given to patients causes problems (in rare cases).

g. Unnecessary back-and-forth discussions by aggrieved customers for minor issues.

h. Pest control is not properly done, leading to insects and rats destroying medicine.

i. Sometimes, due to wrong billing of medicines and/or implants for any reason, a mismatch in the amount collected against the inventory is seen.

j. Monitoring cash transactions.

k. Sometimes medicine strips can't be cut but the patient and their attendants get angry and do not want to take the whole strip.

l. Other miscellaneous issues.

The HOD of the pharmacy is always in contact with the MS/CEO/administrator. Generally, the pharmacy has a zero-error philosophy. All the staff should know their responsibilities towards the hospitals. A store/pharmacy works around the clock every day in the majority of hospitals.

Thoughts for policymakers:

Graduates in hospital administration are not joining stores at senior level mainly because of the following reasons:

Techniques of store management are not taught as specialized subjects, resulting in candidates of graduate level who are not competent to handle stores effectively.

Academic institutions have not thought to consider stores as a profession for hospital management graduates.

Due to modernization and advances in technology, there is a need for policymakers to start including subjects dedicated to stores and store management in hospital management courses. This will give hospital administration graduates an edge over other candidates. If this is implemented, the store department of hospitals will reach the next level in proficiency and will give a new meaning to store management by bringing in professionalism. Also, it would reduce unnecessary costs to the hospital.

Conclusion: A store means money and hence store management requires a professional approach. Material management is one of the integral parts of modern management. Hospital administration graduates should take it as a challenge if given a chance to excel in this field and join as store managers at the senior level.

Lesson 17

Information technology (IT) department

The information technology (IT) department is a very important part of the hospital. Here, non-medicos in the department take care of the entire hospital's information and communication between employees as well as patients. In this department, every executive has IT skills. They are tasked with digitizing billing, admissions, laboratory and diagnostics reports, accounts, finance, pharmacy and biomedical stock, maintenance records, housekeeping records, human resources records, sales and marketing records, reception records, etc. All reports from the laboratories and diagnostic department are communicated to the medical staff through IT networking. The IT department also helps in data collection, storage of patients' admission files in MRD through digital technology.

The IT department directly or indirectly helps in maintaining law and order by checking through footage on the hospital's CCTV system, which gives the security department an additional edge in controlling thefts or hyper aggression, which prevents disruption of order in the hospital premises. Like other departments, the IT department works around the clock.

Some of the common problems the IT department faces are:

a. Sometimes, computers or networks run slowly, which causes delay in registration (OPD/IPD/ admissions/ billing, etc).

b. In rare cases, computers stop working, resulting in a delay in generating reports.

c. CCTV is not operational/functional.

d. Data is not retrieved on demand.

e. Delay in admission/discharge due to rush in hospital/shortage of manpower.

f.   Clerical error in reporting: name/gender/age/address are not written correctly. Sometimes there are spelling mistakes in the discharge paper as well.

g.   Wi-Fi networks stop or don't work properly.

h.   Error in billing and cash collection.

The entire staff of the IT department, like those who handle hardware, software, data entry, videoconferencing, etc, are non-medicos. The IT head is responsible for all IT-related operations and complaints.

The IT head always works in front of the camera and takes almost the entire load of the hospital information related to patients and staff. If any error or fault pertaining to the IT department is detected by end users or by hospital staff and it is brought to the notice of the administrator, the administrator coordinates with the IT head to resolve the issue as soon as possible.

Future Impact of IT in administration:

1.   Due to the fast-changing IT scenario, cloud computing, artificial intelligence, etc, will play a revolutionary role in the health sector. Its application in parking, security, store, billing, appointment, account, laboratories & diagnostics will have a huge impact in the entire administration system and give new concepts in running the hospital. In the near future, even AI-driven robot doctors, nurses, waiters, technicians, etc, which we have not even imagined. Hence the entire administration will be redefined according to time and evolution of science & technology.

2.   In future, all major hospitals will have a chief information security officer (CISO) to maintain the security of the hospital's digital network and prevent ransomware attacks, phishing attacks, data theft, etc.

"The objective of the IT department is to work 24/7/365 days with total devotion, alertness, commitment and ensure that there is no error anywhere." – VBJ

Lesson 18

Medical records department (MRD)

Non-medicos head the MRD. It is one of the most important departments in hospital for taking care of the following:

a. Keeping records of all the patients for a stipulated time and thereafter destroying the file as per standard NABH/NABL protocol. Depending upon hospital policy, for general case files the MRD keeps files for three years, for five years in case of death cases and for medicolegal cases (MLC), records are kept for ten years. MRD also has a condemnation committee, which meets on a regular basis to destroy the records through the shredder machine.

b. Keeping the records of births and deaths of patients, whichever happens in the hospital.

c. Keeping the records of MLC cases.

d. Keeping the record of HIV/dengue or any other contagious/communicable diseases and updating the government databases on these diseases required by the local municipal government.

e. The MRD plays a very important role: ICD 10 Code (International Classification of Disease Tenth Revision) used by all healthcare providers to classify and code all diagnoses and systems, compare and share data used to track health case statics. Maintaining records is very important for research and academic purposes.

f. Receiving all mail on behalf of the hospital for doctors summoned by court on MLC and if called be present with all records of patients.

g. Documentation and attestation in insurance claims cases.

The MRD is also a full-fledged department having spacious storage for records. However, many hospitals have started keeping the records of patients' files in digital mode, which reduces costs on manpower and power generation.

Some of the problems faced by the MRD manager are in amending death and birth certificates, which is very tedious and requires many legal formalities such as Aadhaar card, voter card, identity card, etc, for correction.

The MRD manager directly reports to the medical superintendent but whenever a patient or an attendant brings any problem pertaining to the MRD, the administrator coordinates with the MRD and resolves the issues at the earliest.

The department works only during the day and there is no roster duty for employees.

The motto of the MRD is **"service with compassion"**.

Lesson 19

Kitchen department

The hospital's kitchen department is a very important department. It caters to IPD patients and staff. It is headed by a non-medico who has experience with and previous exposure to hospital catering services. In some hospitals, kitchen and canteen services are outsourced. However, a majority of the hospitals have a full-fledged kitchen department.

The kitchen department has two main tasks:

1. To prepare food for admitted patients and staff on duty.

2. To ensure that the cafeteria has arrangements of fast food and non-alcoholic beverages for OPD patients and their attendants.

The kitchen manager's main tasks are the following:

1. Procuring materials, utensils, and ensuring the storage and preservation of perishable items.

2. Procuring consumable items, like fruits, milk, curd, eggs, etc, on a daily basis.

3. Maintain an inventory of dry rations and non-perishable goods, while keeping a stock of them for at least 15 days.

The store and kitchen manager always remain in touch with the chief dietician for requirements and procurements. If needed, they purchase a range of other things than food items, like chairs, tables, fridges, airconditioners, etc, in consultation with management.

The chief dietician is the head of catering services, and is responsible to provide food and nourishment for the IPD patients, as well as those in the ICU and ward. They must also take care of providing refreshments to blood donors, the preventive check-up area and day-care patients.

Dietician

In hospitals, dieticians are healthcare professionals who are experts in customizing a patient's diet and nutrition during treatment. They know exactly what type of food should be provided to what type of patient.

The main responsibility of the chief dietician are as follows:

1. Ensure the right food for the appropriate patients in all sections of the hospitals. The dietician takes daily rounds (morning and evening) to prepare a list of the total number of diets for patients, the number of soft diets, diabetic diets, non-diabetic diets, etc. The dietician then sends this list to the head cook for the preparation of food.

2. Check the case file of the patient, consult the treating doctor and then fix the diet for patients.

3. To ensure the food served is up to the hospital standard.

4. The dietician must counsel patients at their bedside during their daily rounds.

5. Fixing roster duty for dieticians for the morning and evening shifts.

6. Training of dietician, waiters, cooks, etc, as per NABH guidelines.

7. OPD consultation by a dietician.

There is no night shift for dieticians in the majority of hospitals.

Some common problems a chief dietician faces are:

1. Adulteration in foodgrain, like in rice, pulses, etc.

2. In rare cases, insects and foreign objects, like plastic and metal pieces, are also seen in the food served to patients.

3. Sometimes, there is an error in the diet schedules for diabetic and non-diabetic patients.

4. In rare cases, the quality of the food is found to be substandard.

5. Cold meals are served, which may cause patient dissatisfaction.

6. Sometimes patients want the food against the dietician's advice.

7. Food from outside the hospital is not allowed, but the patient's attendant brings it for them anyway.

8. Other unforeseeable problems.

*[**Note:** Special precaution must be taken for patients who are drowsy and unconscious, or feeding through a tube. For them, special nutrient supplements should be provided according to the doctor's or the dietician's advice and the feeding timetable and the content is strictly monitored.]*

The chief dietician is also a member of the committee where feedback is received from patients every fortnight or every month. They receive vital information from patients, which helps them take corrective measures if required. Feedback is also required to measure the satisfaction level of the patient, which is one of the criteria for ensuring the success and progress of the hospitals.

If any administrative problems, change in diet schedules or any other issue pertaining to diet emerge, then the dietician should immediately take corrective measures. If not manageable, then the dietician should immediately inform the administrative manager or medical superintendent to sort out the problem amicably.

Managing the diet well is very important to keeping patients satisfied, cheerful and upbeat.

The motto of the kitchen department is "ensure satisfaction with a smile."

The administrative manager is not involved in the kitchen's routine operations, but if any problems arise, the administrative manager resolves the issue with the help of the medical superintendent/dietician.

Thought for hospital planners

Hospital management graduates must be taught the following for kitchen management:

1. The kitchen staff must be tested routinely for any infection.

2. Ensure that their personal hygiene is of the highest standard.

3. Monitor perishable and non-perishable items in the kitchen store.

4. Randomly check menu and food for patients if it confirms to the plan as set by the dietician.

Lesson 20

Housekeeping department

This is one of the most important departments of a hospital. It is responsible for maintaining the hygiene and cleanliness of the hospital. A non-medico is the head of the housekeeping department, which is responsible for the cleanliness, hygiene, sanitation, disinfection and mortuary services of the hospital.

Two types of staff work in the housekeeping departments of hospitals:

a. **One shift:** Here, the housekeeping staff arrive early in the morning and open all the departments keeping them neat, clean and dust-free. They work for 8 to 10 hours in the corporate department and outside hospital premises.

b. **Roster shift:** Here, the housekeeping staff work round the clock throughout the year. Their duties are assigned on the hospital's roster in the main building.

The housekeeping department is headed by the housekeeping manager. The chief administration manager is not involved in routine operations. However, whenever a problem arises due to the hospital's housekeeping staff, the administrative manager resolves the problem by taking a progressive and holistic approach.

The housekeeping manager normally faces the following problems:

a. Staff turnover is very high.

b. During festival seasons, getting work from housekeeping staff is troublesome due to frequent absences.

c. A lack of trained housekeeping staff for ICU/wards.

d. Housekeeping staff not wearing masks/gloves while handling waste even after counselling.

e. The staff have a habit of taking lunch or dinner in groups, which may result in delay in attending to patients whenever called or needed.

f.   Keeping contract staff for housekeeping (untrained staff).

g.   Inadequate pest control measures.

h.   Delay in delivering stool pans and urine pots to the patient's bedside.

i.   The mortuary services handled by housekeeping staff sometimes don't follow hospital protocols while handing and/or taking over dead bodies, which may lead to some serious problems.

j.   The housekeeping staff routinely clean the hospital floors using strong disinfectants. Sometimes, they put in more than usual of such chemicals, which may result in burning sensation in the eyes or irritation in the nose and/or throat. Such situations arise primarily because of untrained staff.

Scenario in mortuary services these days:

These days, attendants often want to keep the corpses of their deceased patients in mortuaries for several reasons. Some of them are:

a.   If their blood relatives are staying abroad or out of station.

b.   If attendants want to take the deceased patient for last rites to their hometown, etc, by air, it requires a no-objection certificate from the police station and other formalities pertaining to postmortem and embalming of the body. So, the delay in the formalities causes the mortuary to hold on to the body for longer periods of time.

Mortuary services play a very important role in disposing of dead bodies from the hospital. It is a very emotional affair for family members, and thus the housekeeping manager should personally supervise the process.

'Sharing experience'

a.   Keep in mind that all the valuables should be handed over to their attendant before keeping the dead body in the mortuary.

b.   **Case incidents:**

i. In a rare case, a patient with a head injury, during the operation (decompressive craniotomy), a part of his skull was removed and kept inside the abdomen after slitting it – a standard procedure – and the abdomen was then bandaged. The patient's relatives were briefed by the surgeon about the operation thoroughly. Unfortunately, the patient expired during the operation. However, when the housekeeping staff showed the body to the patient's attendant, one of the relatives got agitated wondering how a brain operation required a bandage on the abdomen. This led to a ruckus. This sensitive issue was brought immediately to the notice of the medical superintendent and chief administrator. The medical superintendent immediately sent ICU doctors to explain to the grieving family about the minutest details of the operation and why it was kept inside the body. This pacified the relatives and the attendant left the place peacefully with the body.

ii. Once, during an electricity outage, the housekeeping staff forgot to file a complaint and the electrician also failed to check the system during a routine check-up. This resulted in the thawing of the bodies kept in the mortuary in subzero temperatures, which led to a foul smell emanating from the facility. This caused a lot of stress on the management for a range of obvious reasons. If any such problem arises, immediately inform the concerned department so that they can carry out repair work and get the mortuary functional immediately. Until then no dead body should be kept there to avoid any untoward incident.

c. Sometimes the housekeeping staff sit together and take food at the mortuary area. *This is totally prohibited.*

The housekeeping manager always manages operational issues in the best interest of the hospital. The staff is also involved in collecting biomedical waste. The housekeeping manager also supervises the disposal of municipal waste to ensure that it is not mixed with biomedical waste and has a blueprint on how to handle this process. The housekeeping staff follow the proper checklist and are always ready to give their 100 per cent in keeping the hospital neat and clean.

Conclusion: The objective of the housekeeping department is "immediate attention and timely execution". If problems are not solved swiftly, they may lead to stress for the hospital authority. Hence, housekeeping managers should be alert, responsible, accountable to work for achieving the goals of the organization.

Thoughts for policymakers:

Graduates from hospital administration are not joining housekeeping as a career option due to the following reasons:

a. University curriculum planners have not thought of housekeeping as a good career option for them, which is in contrast to what has been observed in graduating hotel management, where many graduates join the housekeeping department at the senior level. The hotel industry has always given top priority to housekeeping, even in some 5- to 7-star hotels, housekeeping executives have reached the level of a vice-president.

b. Housekeeping is a very specialized subject. In changing scenarios due to modern and latest technology advancement, housekeeping has now become a benchmark in hotels, malls, hospital industry, etc.

c. Policy planners should provide education and enough material to give career options in housekeeping management. Its importance should not be underestimated in the present. It can even be called a complete science. The hospital housekeeping department should know how to fight the enemy, like pests, insects, fungi, germs and harmful microorganisms, etc, which harm the hospital.

j. Hospital housekeeping is one step ahead of hotel housekeeping or mall housekeeping because the hospital housekeeping staff are in direct contact with the patients. They even help them in private things, like in urination, passing stool, and washing their faecal matter. ii. To relieve severe constipation, the housekeeping staff administers enema (a very personalized care) to patients under the supervision of doctors and nurses.

d. Housekeeping works round the clock throughout the year because a patient's needs in matters such as disposing of waste matter lie on the shoulder of the housekeeping staff.

Due to modernization and advancements in housekeeping, hospital planners must think of a career option for hospital management graduate at the senior level by including specialized subjects on:

a. Municipal waste.

b. Laboratory waste.

c. Radiology film waste

d. E-waste.

e. Dialysis waste.

f. Biomedical waste, like body parts, bone fragments, tissues, blood, etc.

g. Scraps in hospital and disposal procedures.

h. CSSD/laundry waste.

i.   National green tribunal and its role.

j.   Kitchen waste and its disposable plan.

k.   Role of sanitization.

If added, this will definitely benefit the next level of hospital housekeeping and thus help achieve the organization's goals.

Lesson 21

Laundry department

The laundry department is a very important department. This department is headed by a non-medico. Most hospitals have in-house laundry facilities, although in some hospitals it is outsourced. The laundry department has a large storage/ godown for keeping clean clothes as well as a large collection centre for used clothes, linen and other laundry items.

The used clothes, like gowns, aprons, bedsheets, etc are first washed according to the hospital's protocol in the laundry facilities. Then, they are sent to the ironing facilities to make garments presentable and wrinkle free. After washing, the used and infected linen is sent to the CSSD department for sterilization. The waste and infected water is sent to the disinfection tank, where it is treated with chemicals following the hospital's protocols.

The laundry manager faces an excessive workload during the following cases:

a. During peak season.

b. During the rainy and winter season.

c. During disasters.

d. Machines and facilities suffer breakdowns.

e. Lack of adequate pest control.

f. Other unforeseeable circumstances.

The laundry department keeps a reserve stock of clothes for a week or more depending upon the size of the hospital. The laundry department's routine starts around 8am and works in shifts around the clock. The laundry department takes care of all the clothes, bedsheets, pillow covers, blankets, curtains, bedsheets, patient dress, doctor gowns, aprons etc. Even sofas and chairs are washed through hospital protocol and sterilized to be as clean as possible.

The chief administrator does not interfere in the routine work of the laundry department, but if any patient complains about laundry services the manager resolves the issue.

Some problems a laundry manager faces are:

a.   Some clothes are stained due to blood or chemicals.

b.   Some torn clothes, like bedsheets, pillow covers, blankets, etc, are sent to the ward by mistake.

c.   In rare cases, bedbugs are found on blankets or bedsheets due to inadequate pest control.

d.   Other issues.

The laundry department is always in touch with other departments, like housekeeping, CSSD and pathology, to get help and advice to periodically provide clean clothes and garments. The laundry department is headed by the laundry manager, who reports to the medical superintendent.

The administrative manager and medical superintendent supervise the "condemnation" protocol, where torn, stained and old clothes are destroyed.

Conclusion: Patients and patients' attendants are pleased to see a clean environment, including the conditions of the clothes and garments. Thus, the laundry department is a reflection of how much importance a hospital gives to hygiene.

Hospital management graduates must be taught the following on laundry management:

1.   About sluice area, dirty cloth area, clean area, the chemicals used for cleaning.

2.   If laundry services are outsourced, the quality control manager must visit their third-party cleaning facility periodically to ensure if cleaning protocols are followed.

3.   Stain removal processes, staff hygiene, and safe practices, etc.

Lesson 22

Horticulture department

One of the non-medical departments in a hospital is the horticulture department. In this department, the gardener or garden supervisor directly reports to the chief administrator. The horticulture department takes care of all the parks, the plants, and the landscape inside and outside the hospitals.

The gardener, depending upon the season, grows plants to reap and blossom. During festival seasons, the horticulture department puts extra effort to enhance the beauty and aesthetics to ensure that the hospital looks elegant and gives out positive vibes. In some hospitals, gardeners are also responsible for helping make showers with various colours and lighting.

In general, the horticulture department, with the help of the chief administrator, fulfils the requirements needed to maintain a park: fertilizers, seeds, small plants for parks, placing plants inside the hospital corridors, reception area, etc.

The horticulture department only works in the morning shift. Hospitals recruit gardeners through the personnel department. In some hospitals, however, it is outsourced or gardeners do the job in on a daily-wage basis.

The horticulture department follows the rules and regulations of the state horticulture department and the National Green Tribunal. If any problem occurs in this department, then the chief administrator resolves these issues by taking a holistic view. The main job of the horticulture department is to maintain greenery and thus provide fresh air to the hospital's environment.

In some hospitals, a green committee is there to look after and advise the horticulture staff.

Still, an old problem exists in the horticulture department. Hospital planners have not thought about good career options for hospital management graduates in this department.

Suggestion: Hospital planners should provide more information to hospital management graduates about plantation, design, and plants to present an elegant look. Hospital planners should combine the housekeeping and horticulture departments to have a full-fledged department.

Even proper utilization of wastewater or rainwater harvesting systems for the irrigation of the plants, including organic fertilizer decomposed from hospital kitchen waste, dead leaves through sustainable compost techniques should be used in hospitals. The reason is simple: reusing water and using organic fertilizers reduce cost and damage to the environment.

If a hospital management graduate knows enough in subjects on sustainable development, horticulture management and housekeeping management, it will make the hospital a success and a combination of the above will ensure a good career option for hospital management graduates at the senior level. In the hotel industry, housekeeping and horticulture are two major professional wings, which ensure a clean and green environment. Hospitals could do well to follow the hotel industry in this matter.

Future of horticulture department in hospitals:

These days, several big hospitals are working on becoming "green hospitals" for safeguarding the environment. Recycling waste through effluent-treatment plants and adopting sustainable technology, like solar power, will not only keep the environment clean but will also save a significant amount of the hospital's expenditure.

In the coming days, biomedical engineers, horticulture experts, hospital management graduates will have several attractive non-medical careers in the healthcare sector.

"The motto of the horticulture department is to ensure fresh air in and around the hospital, give the facility a cheerful and positive feel through nature and make the establishment environment friendly."
– VBJ

Lesson 23

Security and parking department

The security and parking department has only non-medico staff and it is headed by a non-medico. However, there are some hospitals where the security services are outsourced.

The primary duty of this department is to maintain law and order, traffic and parking in the hospital, which is essential for the safety of the hospital's infrastructure, equipment and all other assets. Therefore, the security and parking department works around the clock throughout the year.

As the department's name suggests, it has two components:

1. Security
2. Parking

Security

Security plays a very important role in the following circumstances:

1. During disasters.
2. During epidemics and pandemics.
3. When VIP patients are admitted.
4. During deaths of influential/VIP patients.
5. If hospital equipment is lost or stolen.
6. During code blue/code black/code violet/code red/code pink.
7. Entry and exit of equipment, instruments, items of the hospital.
8. Parking management and transport area.
9. In the casualty area, ward and ICU for controlling visitors' gathering.

10. CCTV installation in all areas.

11. When visitors to the hospital are carrying arms.

12. Other miscellaneous work.

In most hospitals, ex-servicemen from the military, police, paramedical staff generally head the security department with the help of security officers/security guards.

The security personnel are deployed in two places:

1. **Outside the hospital:** Security personnel are deployed at the entry gate and exit gates, parking/garden areas for smooth parking and peaceful environment.

2. **Inside the hospital:** All the departments such as emergency, ICU, ward, OT, laboratory & diagnostics centre, blood bank, stores, etc.

CCTV cameras are installed in all important departments and locations inside and outside the hospital building to ensure a disciplined and controlled environment and keep a constant watch on people's activities in the premises.

The security department usually intervenes in the following situations:

a. Sometimes, a vehicle's driver brings an injured person to the hospital after hitting the person with his vehicle accidentally. This may cause some friction between the patient's relatives and the driver.

b. Patients who are brought dead, especially if young, can sometimes cause conflict between the dead person's family members and the hospital. Sometimes people from a company or factory bring the patient who is dead and start creating problems as well.

c. Assault on doctors or patients.

d. Suicide cases.

e. Fights between relatives in the hospital.

f. RTA/MLC cases.

g. Cases of theft.

h. Code violet/code pink/heavy rush inside the hospital.

i. Missing patients.

j.   Friction between staff.

k.   Other unforeseen issues.

All the above problems require immediate action. If the head of the security department feels a situation is going out of control, then they should call the police to handle the problem in consultation with the medical superintendent or administration manager.

Observations:

1.   Hospital security is a very challenging assignment but very different from working in the military or police forces, as no drastic action is required as there is no threat from an outside enemy.

2.   Various patients require different kinds of control, like patients with mental illness or psychological problems and hyper-aggressive patients/attendants.

3.   It has been observed that security personnel in hospitals who have had a military or police background have a penchant for strictly adhering to the rules and regulations. This is not exactly what a hospital needs from them. The hospital security personnel must be trained to show a certain degree of flexibility whenever a situation demands.

Case studies:

Incident 1: Once, a depressed patient in OPD suddenly became hyper aggressive and bolted the door of the doctor's chamber from inside when the doctor was with a patient and was about to harm the doctor. The alert guard and staff acted fast and saved the doctor as well as the patient from getting injured.

Incident 2: Once, a depressed patient suddenly jumped from the first floor of the building and sustained serious injuries.

Incident 3: An adult patient went missing from the ward.

These kinds of incidents keep on occurring in hospitals which defence personnel are not familiar with how to handle them.

Incident 4: The standard protocols are always kept in place by security management. Only persuasion, compassion and counselling are required to solve most issues. Thus security requires empathy, common sense, compassion and logical handling when dealing with colleagues, patients and visitors.

The hospital security system may be renamed as the hospital "peacekeeping force" for the following reasons:

a. This will give a clear message to the general public that the hospital peacekeeping force is there for their help, the safety of staff and property and is in no way against any individual, as long as they are obeying the rules.

b. Provide the security personnel with advanced gadgets and backup with proper training exclusively for hospital work. This will make a qualitative change in the security department.

Parking

Non-medical or support staff manage the parking areas. There are three types of parking facilities:

1. Ground-level parking.
2. Underground/basement parking.
3. Multi-level parking

Depending upon the size of the hospital, parking is divided into two categories:

1. Staff parking.
2. Parking for patients/attendants.

Staff parking.

1. Parking of hospital staff of two wheelers/bicycles.
2. Parking of hospital staff of four wheelers.

For patients/attendants.

1. For two wheelers/bicycles.
2. For four wheelers.

Miscellaneous: Temporary three wheelers/four wheelers which are hired for picking up and dropping off patients do not require any fixed parking space.

For all the above parking facilities, a dedicated workforce is required to handle such a huge and complex task.

Parking managers who handle the parking area may face the following difficulties:

a. Theft of vehicles.

b.   Loss of valuables from the vehicle.

c.   Someone hits the parked vehicles.

d.   Someone parks a vehicle in front of another vehicle, blocking the way.

The parking manager always remains in contact with the chief administrative manager to ensure the smooth functioning of a hospital's parking services. If the end users complain, then only the chief admin manager resolves the issue. Reviews are conducted either once a fortnight or on a monthly basis to check the effectiveness of the parking arrangement.

Parking is a challenging assignment for those who handle it. It requires proper management techniques and careful usage of space to handle huge gatherings of vehicles in a specific area with limited space.

Parking in hospitals is a headache during pandemics, epidemics, disasters and even sometimes during the death of a family member of some popular person as a lot of people assemble at the hospital.

Advices:

a.   *The parking staff must follow a checklist provided by parking managers.*

b.   *Parking staff must be courteous and polite while dealing with emotional patients/attendants.*

c.   *Parking staff should never take law & order in their own hands. If any problems arise, they should report them to their superiors and the security officers.*

d.   *A CCTV system should be installed in the entire parking area to keep a constant vigil.*

[Note: If a patient or attendant comes in a car and starts to honk, never shout at them. Be polite and courteous don't reply back. Never argue with them and, instead, focus on how to resolve the matter. If you can't handle or resolve the issue yourself, call your senior.]

Observation:

In spite of people's changing lifestyle and advancement in transport management, age-old practices continue. Hence, traffic management within the hospital premises remains a major challenge.

Maintaining a parking facility on a contractual basis or with unorganized sectors' workforce or with the hospital's employees requires a total review of the current methodology of parking and traffic management in the hospital. Sometimes during peak hours morning and evening OPD, there is total chaos. Until now, hospital planners have not focused on parking, and there are many issues that would not occur if traffic management had been more carefully planned.

Hence hospital planners should keep qualified/experienced people to handle parking issues carefully with the help of latest gadgets.

A hospital management graduate must be taught about parking and traffic management in a hospital. With proper training and a scientific approach, solutions can be devised for monitoring and managing traffic.

Thoughts for hospital planners:

Changing times bring new challenges. In order to tackle new challenges, hospital planners must do research on security and parking in hospitals periodically and include their findings and recommendations in hospital management courses.

Lesson 24

Transport department

Non-medicos work and run the hospital transport department. The transportations are of mainly three types:

1. Ambulance: It transports sick or injured people to and from the hospital. They carry oxygen cylinders and emergency medicines with paramedical staff.

2. ACLS ambulance (advanced cardiac life support): This type of ambulance has doctor/nurse/paramedical staff, an emergency kit, oxygen cylinders and defibrillator, pulse oximeter and all emergency equipment for transporting patients to hospitals.

3. Passenger transport (bus/car etc) for doctors/staff/ management.

4. Miscellaneous:

    i. If the distance is too long between the parking lot and a specialty area, the hospital provides free transportation. These are done by vehicles that can carry between 9 to 12 patients/passengers within a short time.

    ii. The transport department has a hearse, which is usually a van to take a dead body from the hospital mortuary to the home of the dead person. Also, when dealing with MLC cases, the corpse has to be transported to a postmortem facility. In some hospitals, hearse services are outsourced.

It has been observed that sometimes attendants want to take the bodies of their departed ones to their native place for last rites by air. Here, the administrative manager coordinates with the police department to get a no-objection certificate (NOC) for them. At the same time, the transport manager apprises the patient's attendant with embalming protocols before shifting the body to the airport. An NOC and embalming are mandatory for shifting a dead body by air.

Routine problems, instructions, calls, shifting and execution are all catered to by the transport department with the help of the transport manager.

The entire fleet of vehicles is controlled by the transport manager (a non-medico) to take care of patients and staff. In exceptional cases, a "green corridor" is provided by the state government agency to bring the patients from an affected area to the hospital site in the shortest possible time. Here, hospital staff liaison with the government and police officers to carry out the mission.

Some problems a transport manager can face with ambulances are:

1. In emergency services, sometimes a wrong address is provided that results in a delay in an ambulance reaching its destination.

2. The ambulance meets with a road accident.

3. Excessive traffic slows the ambulance.

4. Sometimes, most of the ambulances are sent for fuelling, which results in a shortage of ambulances until they return.

5. Maintenance of ambulances and vehicles takes too long.

6. Outsourced vehicles/ambulances are not available on time.

7. In some rare cases, emergency medicines are not available in the ambulance, or even oxygen cylinders are not functional.

8. Other unforeseen issues.

Advice: Follow the checklist before leaving the hospital.

A hospital ambulance is available around the clock every day of the year.

The administration manager is not involved in the day-to-day operations of the transport management. If an end user or someone else brings any problems related to transport to his notice, then the administrator will sort out any problems.

The transport department also has a vehicle maintenance workshop in some hospitals. Otherwise, in most hospitals, the transport maintenance services are outsourced or the hospital has an annual maintenance contract with automobile workshops.

Ambulance services usually get duty calls from the following places:

1. Directly on mobile or on landline from the reception.

2. Information received through casualty area/ward/ICU for DOR/ LAMA/referral/discharge patients/outsource diagnostics tests.

3. Information is directly sent to ambulance service personnel on their mobiles.

All the staff work as a team to provide the best health care facility to patients.

The mottos of ambulance and hearse services are

1. To ensure urgent medical services by bringing patients to hospital

2. To shift the patient as needed either referral, an outsourced investigation, taking them home or even for postmortem (upon death).

Some points to remember:

1. For emergency transportation of organs for transplant and sometimes even important medicines from one station to another station for patients, a "green corridor" is provided to reach safely within a short time. Here, a great deal of communication and coordination is required to obtain the desired results.

2. During disaster management, the hospital transport system has a very important role in bringing sick and injured people to the hospital under great pressure. It needs deft handling to smoothly run the transporting operations, which includes transporting doctors and staff to the hospital from their residence.

3. During epidemics and pandemics, ambulance services are not just for patients. Vehicles are also required to ferry doctors and staff for which additional permission is required from the local administration. The drivers and support staff also need to take special precautions to deal with doctors and other staff during transportation.

4. During curfews and lockdowns, the hospital transport services become essential services, requiring a great deal of coordination with state government machinery. The transport manager plays a very important role in handling this.

5. Even parking is paired with the transport department to handle more than 400 vehicles a day in a large hospital. Handling such a vast amount of traffic requires careful logistics and management. A policy planner should add this to hospital management graduate courses, it will open up a number of job opportunities.

6. Due to advances in transportation, these days air ambulances are also hired or purchased by large hospitals to shift patients from one site to another site for better medical attention.

7. Due to advances in IT/artificial intelligence and continuous upgradation to ambulances and other vehicles, the transport system, its way of operation and transport facilities will see big changes in the near future. For this, hospital management graduates with transport management skills will be better equipped to handle transport departments efficiently.

Advice: Hospital staff must be trained to transport patients from multistorey buildings when there is a power outage or lift become dysfunctional. This is to ensure that the patient, their attendants, and the hospital staff don't face any incident, such as an injury or a mishap, while shifting the patients from one floor to another.

Thought for policymakers:

The transport department in hospitals is very important. Handling transport and logistics should be done by a senior management.

Hospital management graduates with hospital experience don't even think of joining as transport managers. This is because hospital management graduates are not taught about hospital transport management. Just one chapter or a few details of ambulances are being taught. Hence, there is a treasure of untapped opportunities for hospital management graduates to join the transport department.

Due to advances in transportation and ambulance services, it has become an upcoming field with a vast scope. Hospital management graduates should be taught how to handle transportation with modern technology, such as managing transportation through GPS and use of digital map services, like Google Maps, to help the transport system run smoothly.

"Hospital management graduates with experience in transportation will be better suited than regular transport managers because transportation is becoming a tech-based specialized task." – VBJ

Lesson 25

Maintenance and biomedical department

Non-medical professionals manage the maintenance and biomedical department. The department is headed by a chief engineer.

The department is divided into two parts:

1. Core maintenance unit.
2. Biomedical unit.

Core maintenance unit:

Hardware, infrastructure, rainwater drainage system, water storage, electricals, airconditioning, lifts, plumbing, etc, come under the core maintenance unit. Some of the employees working in this unit are engineers with degrees, diploma holders and with ITI background. Unskilled work is also a part of the engineering team where support staff work as contract labourers on temporary contracts. This unit employs staff who work around the clock by rotation.

In some hospitals, the work of the core maintenance unit is outsourced but in most cases, this unit is a part of the hospital itself.

The entire infrastructure of the hospital is maintained by the engineering team. Maintenance problems are noted at the complaint cell every day and hospital staff and patient's attendants record their grievances as well. The complaint cell works around the clock to resolve all the complaints within the stipulated time. The complaint register is checked by the chief maintenance engineer every day to keep control over the engineering team and to provide a smooth and complaint free environment.

Most of the complaints this unit receives are related to power, airconditioners, fridges, coolers, televisions, plumbing, drainage system, computers, generators, voltage fluctuations, geysers, call bells, telephones, drinking water, RO water, etc. They mostly come from the ward, ICU, OT, kitchen department, laundry department, dialysis department, IT department, CSSD, etc. It is the duty of the engineering department to ensure all these things run smoothly so that the hospital can provide care without hindrance.

The motto of the core maintenance unit is *"work around the clock"* to ensure:

1. Timely completion of work.

2. Timely renewal of annual maintenance contracts.

3. Focus on measures to prevent breakdown/outage of machinery/ electricity.

4. Ensuring the safety of employees, machines and property.

5. To look for cost-effective solutions.

Mock drills: Mock drills are also one of the most important protocols of the maintenance unit, which should be repeated every three months. Mock drills for fire and disaster are regular features to keep the maintenance unit alert and able to work in all emergency situations.

The chief maintenance engineer is also a member of the feedback committee which reviews feedback from the patients every fortnight or every month. It is a tool to measure the patient's satisfaction as well as to get feedback on the work of the maintenance and biomedical department.

The administrator is not involved in the routine workings of the maintenance department but if any problem occur, they should immediately discuss it with the person concerned to sort out the problem swiftly.

Biomedical unit

The biomedical unit also has non-medico staff. The biomedical engineer heads this department. It is a very challenging unit and is the livewire of hospital services.

The biomedical engineering team takes care of all equipment and machine used for patients, such as MRI machine, CT-scan machine, x-ray machine, ventilator, ultrasound, catheterization labs, CSSD plant, equipment in the pathology lab, non-invasive diagnostic lab, physiotherapy equipment, pulse oximetry, ECG, EEG, OPG, oxygen plants, etc.

The biomedical department work around the clock and faces the following problems:

1. Breakdown of important machines used for MRI, CT scans, catheterization lab, etc.

2. Delays in repair work. It may be due to spare parts not being provided in time by suppliers, and implementing contingencies takes more time.

3. Preventive measures and checklists are not followed, causing a breakdown.

Two kinds of machine management are carried out in the biomedical department:

1. Machines and equipment are under an annual maintenance contract.

2. Machines and equipment are not under an AMC, instead the hospital has in-house mechanisms for repairing equipment or getting them repaired from the market.

The biomedical engineer solves these routine problems related to biomedical equipment and machines. If they cannot resolve an issue on their own, the engineer immediately coordinates with the medical superintendent to deal with it.

Conclusion: The chief administration manager does not handle the day-to-day working of the biomedical unit. However, whenever any issues emerge, they coordinate with the biomedical engineer to help resolve them.

The motto of the biomedical department is to work around the clock, smoothly, efficiently, and safely. Biomedical managers also provide checklists, calibration methods and preventive measures to help avoid accidents in hospitals, playing a vital role in ensuring the hospital runs smoothly.

Future:

The world is changing at a rapid pace. It is not the same as it was 500 years ago and neither it will be the same as it is today in the future. The world will face new challenges that will arise out of climate change, natural calamities, human-nature conflict, changes in the lifestyle of people and new diseases.

To overcome these challenges, hospital planners will have no option but to adopt new technology in infrastructure, civil, mechanical, electronic, IT and energy sectors. For this, the maintenance department will also have to be in sync with the trends and demands of the challenges. This will also result in hospitals employing engineers, workers and consultants who are trained in new technologies and have a reasonable understanding of future trends and challenges.

"The safety of the employees and patients while handling machinery and equipment is very important, and it is the maintenance and biomedical department that helps ensure it." – VBJ

Lesson 26

Reception department

The reception department is the mirror of the hospital. This department is headed by non-medicos. The role of the reception department are as follows :

1. To attend to both incoming and outgoing calls for doctors, staff and patients/patients' attendants.

2. To provide correct information whenever any person inquires.

3. To carry out orders from seniors to announce disaster, mock drill, code red, code violet and code pink

4. To have "May I help You" counters to guide patients and their attendants and also address their grievances. They also pass messages on to other concerned departments to do needful.

5. To have a data bank of all important numbers of doctors, management, staff and admitted patients including police stations, police officers/government agency/TPA and panel companies/officials and office numbers.

6. To announce through the public address system in case of any urgent information needs to be shared with all.

7. To immediately transfer calls to the transport department whenever requests for ambulances are made.

The head of the reception department ensures round-the clock availability of staff in the three shifts. The administrative manager does not interfere in the day-to-day operations of the reception department, but whenever any person comes with a complaint to the reception, the receptionist conveys it to the administrative manager or concerned department to resolve the issue.

Words of caution:

1. If phone calls come from outside inquiring about an admitted patient's condition, never ever inform the prognosis of the patient telephonically just by getting his or her name. Sometimes more than one patient with the same name is admitted at the same time. Therefore, ask more details, like the patient's father's/mother's name, age, address, etc. When sure, transfer the call to the treating doctor or concerned department, who will then brief the caller about the patient's condition.

2. If the reception receives a call of a threat, like a bomb in the hospital premises, don't panic, but don't take it as a hoax call by default. Note down the caller's number and immediately report it to the security department and other hospital authorities.

3. If a female receptionist receives an obscene call, note down the caller's number and immediately report it to the security department and the head of the reception department.

"The objective of the reception department is to maintain goodwill of the hospital with a mission for speedy redressal of issues." – VBJ

Lesson 27

Marketing department

Most non-medico employees in a hospital work for the marketing department of the hospital. These days, hospital management graduates are also taking the initiative to join the marketing department for two reasons:

1. Unlimited growth opportunities.

2. Attractive perks.

Those who work in the marketing department range from multitasking staff to specialist executives, like business development. They are all are from non-medical background and employed in various marketing roles such as:

1. Getting government, semi-government, public sector, private sector organizations into the hospital's panel for the treatment of their employees and their dependants.

2. For insurance panel/TPA work.

3. Promotion of hospitals, such as advertising in newspapers, electronic media, privilege cards, advertisement of camps, CME, preventive health check-up camp, public lecture on prevention of disease, cause and treatment.

4. Arrange news conferences in and outside of the hospital.

5. Marketing staff sometimes help in obtaining a good consultant from the outside.

6. Medical tourism, which is a new concept of bringing patients from other countries.

7. Bill recovery.

8. Opening of clinics in schools and panel companies

9. Make strategy for home collection of samples.

10. New concept video consultation, e-marketing through digital media, such as YouTube, Facebook, WhatsApp, etc.

11. Miscellaneous work if any, as per management requirements.

Conclusion:

Marketing is an essential function to ensure a demand for cost-effective health care services with modern facilities, hence the need for focused investment.

In the healthcare industry, marketing personnel must know that the hospital industry is not a product-oriented sector, which requires promotion like the FMCG industry. It is an emotional service sector where patients get treated by doctors and "service with empathy" is the USP, and one has to balance between the humane and commercial approaches. Hence the marketing team always takes a cautious approach during presentation.

It is an age-old saying that doctors run the hospitals. However, with the passage of time, the latest way to have a complete package for the hospital is to build a brand – a key to its success. Thus the marketing team works relentlessly on building a brand for reliable and trustworthy hospital chains.

The administrator has very little say in the day-to-day activities of the marketing department. However, the administrator helps coordinate and liaisons with marketing personnel if any assistance is required from the hospital.

Often, the administration seeks the help of marketing personnel regarding TPA/panel patients – whenever it is needed – for things, like legal statutory requirement from panel, an extension of a panel patient's treatment as per doctor's advice, obtaining approval from a government agency for costly procedures, implants, medicine, chemotherapy drugs, etc.

Thus, the administrator is always in touch with marketing personnel to sort out all legal statutory requirements to arrange the best medical treatment for panel patients.

The head of marketing is always in contact with the MS/chief administrator, and formulates strategies based on feedback from management, patients and patient attendants.

> *"Patients coming from other hospitals as LAMA/DOR/referral or from panel companies require special analysis from the marketing department. They should also make strategies to focus on other areas and panel companies from where footfall of patients is less." - VBJ*

Lesson 28

Quality department

The quality department is the master controller as well as the enforcer of the rule book/constitution of the hospital. The head of the quality department is a medico, who reports to the medical superintendent.

This department is also responsible for charting standard operating procedures for the various departments of the hospital.

The quality department helps in getting certification from the NABH and NABL standards, which is the benchmark for a hospital's accreditation. A high accreditation gives the hospital an advantage in getting privileges from the TPA, corporations, public sector undertakings, state and central governments regarding the formulation of charges.

The quality department works on mission, vision, quality policy, hospital organogram, scope of services, hospital committee, registration policy and procedure, admission policy and procedure, management of bed and resources, transfer and referral of patient, patient initial assessment policy, policy of in-house referral, LAMA policy, colour codes (blue, red, violet, pink), etc.

The subject and content of the quality department set by the NABL and NABH is so vast that an entire book can be written on it. The HOD of the quality department always updates on the latest additions of accreditations to staff and conducts fortnightly or monthly meetings of various committees, like disaster committee, quality and assurance committee, etc, to upgrade the knowledge of the staff continuously.

Hospital planners and academics must also think of broadening the career options of upcoming hospital management graduates. Some of the suggestions are as follows:

Suggestions:

1. Quality management is an upcoming profession. Hospital planners and academicians must encourage hospital management graduates by adding a detailed syllabus about the quality department as set by the NABH, NABL, etc, so that when hospital management graduates leave the university they can take up a job in the quality department.

2. Government of India and state government educational planners still have not thought of providing job opportunities in upcoming national and state health programmes for hospital management graduates.

The introduction of National Health Policy 2017 for universal access to good quality healthcare services and the subsequent launch of Ayushman Bharat had two components:

i.   Health and wellness centre to provide comprehensive primary healthcare.

ii. The Pradhan Mantri Jan Arogya Yojana seeks to provide health cover to 10.74 crore poor and vulnerable families with up to ₹5 lakh per family per year for secondary and tertiary hospitalization.

Apart from the above two, the "mohalla clinic (neighbourhood clinic)" initiative by the Delhi government is also a good programme, which caters to all sections of people living in Delhi. These clinics provide free medicines and treatment.

Both the central and many state governments have various healthcare schemes for the underprivileged, poor, and rural/adivasi population of the country. These are yet to be properly publicized so the schemes can reach those people for whom they have been launched. The primary health centres, community health centres, and many more state-run programmes require a review and fresh focus to make everyone know how to reach the government facilities and avail the schemes.

In other words, the central and state governments, healthcare sectors and NGOs should work to provide good career opportunities for hospital management graduates to serve their country and help uplift the nation's health.

3. It is observed that hospital management graduates have not been provided with enough facilities and career options to join in research activities in academia. This anomaly must be fixed and those who are studying hospital management must be encouraged to do research work.

Conclusion: Health planners and university scholars must include the above subjects and programmes in detail in the curriculum to encourage hospital management graduates to explore untapped areas of career opportunity, including jobs in research and quality departments.

Lesson 29

Feedback panel

Feedback mechanisms are a very important tool to gauge the satisfaction level of the hospital's patients. The medical superintendent chairs the feedback committee, and on either a biweekly or monthly basis feedback is collected and compiled by staff. The committee members consist of the chief administrator, chief dietician, chief maintenance engineer, housekeeping manager, security chief, personnel manager, billing manager, nursing superintendent and head of the laboratory & diagnostics, as well as the chief of the quality department.

A suggestion box is kept in each and every area and patients are encouraged to share their feedback and put it in the box. On a fixed date, senior managers of the different departments gather and one by one information from the feedback forms is studied and if required, they make a phone call to the concerned person for more inputs. Sometimes, they write to the patients regarding action taken or by thanking them for their suggestions and information on the feedback form.

Some common complaints are related to issues like blankets and warmers not being provided during winter, toilets not being properly maintained, too much noise, inadequate pest control, doctors arriving late, the doctors not spending enough time with the patient, misbehaviour staff, malfunctioning civil works, neglectful security staff, TPA grievances, extra bill charges about diet and food management, etc.

Sometimes, some amusing things are mentioned in the feedback form by small children, like chocolates and ice cream were not given to them or the doctor was not smiling when the child came for the consultation.

The feedback form is a vital source and can be used as an important administrative tool for proper analysis of a patient's grievances, complaints, suggestions and to take corrective measures.

The management should take all feedback seriously and monitor them carefully to help the hospital grow. Often, suggestions and corrective measures are implemented based on patient feedback.

Each and every department designs the feedback form according to their specialty, like the following:

1. OPD Feedback

2. IPD feedback

3. Lab and diagnostic feedback

4. physiotherapy feedback

5. Blood bank feedback

6. Dental feedback

The size and the specialty of the hospital are also taken into account when designing forms.

On the basis of feedback received from the hospital, the quality department formulates patients' satisfaction statistics and data for NABH, NABL and ISO accreditation purposes. At least 80 per cent of the feedback forms from all the departments that deal with patients have to be analysed for accuracy, for which the floor manager, sister in charge, ward manager and administrator plays a very important role .

Conclusion: The feedback form is an essential tool for monitoring the level of patient satisfaction in each hospital. The administrative manager ensures that each department gets the patients and/or their attendants to fill their feedback forms. This helps to form a true picture of the hospital from the perspective of the patients.

Note: In some hospitals, chairman or managing director or the owner of the hospital keeps the keys of feedback box handy and opens it regularly on a fixed date.

Lesson 30

Personnel/Human resource department

The personnel or the human resource (HR) department of hospitals is headed by non-medico professionals. The personnel manager has the following responsibilities:

1. Recruitment of both medical and non-medicos personnel.

2. Handle disbursement of salary and expenses.

3. Manage PF/ESI/welfare benefits.

4. Handle leave/LTC management/disbursement for eligible staff.

5. Handle induction appraisal, review, reward, increment, promotion, posting and job transfers.

6. Organize skill development and training as well continuous medical education programme (CME) for doctors, nurses, paramedical, technicians, and staff.

7. Handle the suspension, penalty and general disciplinary actions against any employee after a domestic enquiry. In particular, the internal complaint committee is there to prevent, prohibit and redress any sexual harassment,

8. Maintain a databank of staff with both past and present employees as well as backup candidates

9. Discharge corporate social responsibilities by execution in the relevant projects.

10. Manage contract labour staff, and ensure their benefits and availability.

11. Manage employee life cycle – from appointment till retirement/ resignation.

12. Manage miscellaneous/urgent issues pertaining to the department.

The HR department aids the management in the appointment of the medical superintendent/chief administrator – and the management in turn helps and guides personnel managers in recruiting suitable candidates for hospitals.

The staff is hired after screenings, interviews and written examinations. To help them adapt, the hired candidates are aided by the HR department through an induction programme where they are briefed about the hospital's various specialties by all the department heads. The focus is on the vision, mission, quality, culture and ethos of the hospital, which helps the workforce build confidence as they integrate with the hospital environment.

The personnel manager faces the following problems:

1. There is a high turnover of nurses, IT and housekeeping staff, and keeping backups is always a challenge.

2. Verification of Class 4 employees from the police station is always a headache as turnover is high, and sometimes they leave without giving any notice to the hospital.

3. Employees leave without notice.

4. Staffers want to be transferred to a more favourable posting.

5. Gratuity/bond issues, if any.

6. In the event of the death of any employee, settling claims and closing their file.

7. Strike, labour issue, staff infighting and unrest among employees due to various issues.

8. Sudden resignation from duties/mass resignation of employees.

9. Managing outsourced resources.

10. Conspiracy by employees against the hospital management to damage reputation.

Thought for policymakers:

Very few students from hospital administration join the HR department despite human resources management being one of the most challenging and enduring professions. Academic institutions should provide specialized courses on this subject in the students' final year as this would open up a good career option for them.

If hospital management graduates join the HR department, it will improve the quality of how hospitals are managed. If they have the basic knowledge of the hospital business, organizational structure, recruitment process, etc, they can recruit new staff for the hospital professionally by better screening their biodata, conducting interviews, etc. Therefore, it is the call of the hour to introduce study modules that would include how to select, induct, designate and manage new staff.

This will also give them an edge over other candidates who aspire to join the HR department.

Conclusion: The personnel department is one of the prominent employment options for hospital administration graduates, and the sooner they grasp these opportunities, the better they will be. Now, due to research and modern advances of technology in the HR department, hospital management graduates can join the HR department as senior positions, just as they do in the hotel industry, where hotel management graduates with a specialization in HR and MBA join as HR manager and have a successful career.

"Never sit idle on a challenge or issue that requires immediate attention. Think and analyse. Refer to the SOPs and act with utmost care, concern and caution." – VBJ

PART – II

From the administrator's desk

The aim of this part of the book is to highlight the challenges the administrator faces while working in a hospital and how to tackle those challenges.

Lessons 1 to 6 discuss administrative challenges, case studies, learning tools, dos and don'ts and advice/suggestions on how to work more efficiently. The aim is to help an aspiring hospital administrator to become a multitasking manager who always leads from the front without disturbing the hospital's ecosystem.

*[**Note:** Some cases and incidents discussed in this part of the book are imaginary and hypothetical in nature. The objective is to keep focus only on the administrative challenges.]*

"Face the situation confidently to handle all problems." – VBJ

Lesson 1

Safeguarding hospital's interests

Based on my experience as a non-medical professional, I can say there is a thin line differentiating the responsibilities of the medical superintendent and the chief administrator. I have observed that on the ground, the duties of both the officers can overlap as they work to sort out problems.

The ultimate goal of both officers is to safeguard the interests of the hospital and solve problems by taking a 360-degree view.

The medical superintendent is the ultimate authority of the hospital, but the chief administrator's role and responsibilities are not to be underestimated. They both work almost around the clock because even if they are at home or on leave, the hospital staff continuously seek their advice and instructions over the phone, texting apps and emails.

Due to industrialization, commercialization and rapidly growing corporate culture, hospitals are also witnessing a great change in management ethics. Hospital planners and entrepreneurs are promoting employees or hiring for posts that are usually seen in the corporate sector, like the posts of CEO, COO, president, vice-president, group director, directors, etc. The idea of appointing people directly to senior positions in the healthcare industry may be due to the following reasons:

1. Promoters starting hospital chains for expansion of their brand.

2. Upgrading the facilities and infrastructure of existing hospitals.

3. Going public by offering shares in stock markets.

4. For diversification, like medical tourism, collaborating with other hospitals, merging with other hospitals, etc.

5. Other miscellaneous reasons.

Hypothetical scenarios:

Now, let me discuss three imaginary incidents that could happen to any big hospital.

Incident 1:

Once an IT employee was assigned to help the billing department in the OPD as a billing executive. Taking advantage of the work pressure staff in the department face, the person exploited the loopholes in the billing system and started embezzling the refund money of one or two bills per day. The OPD manager didn't once doubt the billing executive's intentions and he kept on authorizing the latter's vouchers in good faith. This continued for three years, during which the billing executive managed to siphon off ₹2.8 lakh. This came to an end when he was caught by the hospital's vigilance.

Action taken thereafter:

The hospital recovered ₹2.80 lakh from the scamming billing executive and his services were terminated. Additionally, appropriate legal action was taken against him.

Observations:

1. The IT head did not deploy any person for a surprise visit to check on the billing executive's work.
2. The accounts section didn't verify or check the refund rule book. Every day, the same person was coming and getting cash refunds, but the cashier failed to suspect any foul play.
3. The security staff were not checking the CCTV footage of the billing department or the cashier's cabin regularly.
4. The OPD manager kept on signing the vouchers in good faith and failed to follow the checklist for managing refunds. This resulted in the crime under various sections of the Indian Penal Code.
5. The OPD manager was suspended for 30 days.
6. The administrator who had signed the bill, which came from the OPD manager, without crosschecking had his increment delayed by six months.

Root-cause findings:

1. The checklist or circular* for OPD refund was not implemented.

2. The account section didn't verify/crosscheck why the same person was taking refunds almost every day.

[*A refund circular states many clauses under which money is refunded to a patient. The OPD manager must see the patient's bill and only if satisfied that it is a fit case for refund under the circular's clauses, he/she signs the voucher and sends it to the accounts department. Then the head of the OPD and accounts department signs it for approval according to the refunding protocol for completing the refund process.]

Incident 2:

A billing clerk in the dental OPD made a duplicate bill book and started issuing bills from this fake bill book to illiterate patients and/or their attendants who had little or no understanding of such things. This way, the billing clerk managed to make an average of ₹10,000 per month by scamming patients. This went for a few months until he was caught by the hospital's vigilance by sheer chance.

Action taken thereafter:

The management terminated the billing clerk's services and took appropriate legal action against him.

Root-cause findings:

1. No surprise inspections were carried out by the accounts department/collection officers.

2. The dental OPD manager was in the dark, because he was not competent enough to detect the fraud.

Incident 3:

Once, a 46-year-old male came to get the Covid-19 RT-PCR test done on him. After showing his Aadhar card, the billing clerk took a photocopy of the same. After entering the person's information based on his Aadhaar card, the clerk issued him a bill of ₹1,600 for the test.

The report, which came on the next day, showed that he was Covid-19 positive. However, the anxious patient was shocked to see his age on the report as 16 instead of 46. He immediately called the reception, and the receptionist connected him to the administrator. The administrator first listened to the person's complaint. He then apologized and requested him to give him a few minutes to look into the matter.

The administrator then talked to the billing and laboratory department to understand what caused the exact reason for the error, which was found to be clerical. The administrator called the patient and briefed him about the hospital's system. He told the patient that a unique code is always generated on a particular test and a sticker is pasted on the sample vial as well as on the physical bill itself. The test was performed properly and the result was 100 per cent correct and there was no foul play. Since the patient was intelligent and educated, with some knowledge on how hospitals work, he did not overreact.

The administrator also called him to the hospital and took him to a doctor. He was also given a new report which showed his correct age and assured him that such incidents would not happen in the future.

Root-cause findings:

1. The billing clerk did not crosscheck while giving the bill.
2. At the testing area, the public relations officer had called him just by name and did not check his age.
3. The lab technician just called the patient by name and performed the test, and did not crosscheck.

To sum it up, of the three hospital employees who had seen the bill, no one detected the error.

Action taken thereafter:

The management deducted a day's salary from the billing clerk who made the first mistake. However, the others were let off with a verbal reprimand.

Tips for the administrator:

1. Never forget to look beyond the surface of every issue. Think and analyse the problem and always refer to the standard operating procedure. Implement circulars/SOPs with utmost care, concern and caution.
2. One needs to in his/her mind that the higher they climb the hierarchical ladder, the hospital's management will delegate more

power to them, including financial powers, and delegate them on routine duties. Never sign any document or bills without making sure of its authenticity, it has correct details, etc, solely based on good faith or due to lack of time or loss of focus. It is better to be cautious than repent later.

Thought for policymakers:

Hospital and academic planners have so far not put enough emphasis on training hospital management graduates on how to locate such faults. The hospital management graduate must also be taught about how to detect and stop corruption, forgery and theft.

Lesson 2

Tackling unexpected issues

The job of the hospital administration is full of challenges. Every day the administrator faces new challenges, new issues, and sometimes unexpected and strange questions and logic by the patients and/or their attendants. Hospital administrators must understand the gravity of the subject and problems faced by the grieving attendants with composure and try to solve all their issues with empathy and by taking into account all factors.

Unexpected issues present themselves in a hospital all the time and they never go away. If not tackled immediately, those problems become unnecessarily complex issues, which requires the intervention of senior management.

Let us now see some of the administration problems administrators face with four completely imaginary case studies.

Case study 1:

A patient was admitted on a case plan by a haematologist. The doctor saw the patient in the OPD and asked the patient to get admitted at 6am on a particular date. The patient came as per the plan and was admitted on that date at 6am. However, no consultant doctor saw the patient until 2pm. This made the patient attendant ask the ward manager why the hospital was not starting the treatment.

As no one was able to answer the attendant's questions, the attendant started shouting and the situation got out of control. Only then the information was sent to the administrative manager. The administrative manager intervened and probed the matter. He found that the pharmacy did not stock the medicine required for the treatment as it was a costly drug. Secondly, the pharmacy sent someone to buy the medicine in that morning only. The hospital administrator apologized to the attendant for the delay and assured them that the problem would be dealt with soon. Meanwhile, the person dispatched to buy the medicine returned at

2.30pm, and within half an hour, the patient's treatment started in day care. The patient left after the treatment around 6pm in stable condition.

Thanks to the administrative manager's intervention, the patient went home satisfied.

Now, let's analyse the root cause of the issue.

Why was he admitted when the medicine was not available?

The findings were:

1. The RMO at casualty called the consultant before admission. The consultant just told him to "follow the advice" mentioned on the prescription and disconnected the call. Following this, the RMO recommended the casualty manager to admit the patient, who then admitted the patient in the day-care facility.

2. The casualty manager arranged a bed in the day care, but no one informed him that the required drug was not available. *[**Note:** This happens in rare cases.]*

3. The day-care in charge and nurses kept on reminding the consultant, pharmacy and ward manager about the delay in getting the medicine, but no one paid any heed.

4. The pharmacist said the medicine was too costly to keep in stock and is only provided on demand.

[Note: This also shows that the drug formulary was not implemented. A therapeutics panel comprising pharmacist, physicians, surgeons from various medical specialties to run the hospital pharmacy makes the drug formulary. In this case the drug was not available by pharmacy due to a fear of cost and chance of expiry. All drugs listed in the drug formulary should be available, but in special cases where any doctor wants something new, the requested medicine or implant should be passed through the drug formulary committee for the patient's benefit and so that there is transparency in the pharmacy's purchase.]

This also shows that the chain of communication failed at:

1. At the casualty end.

2. At the consultant's end.

3. At the pharmacy's end.

4. At the day-care facility's end.

Observation: If the doctor would have briefed the pharmacy, the OPD and casualty managers about the medicine in advance, the patient would have received the treatment in time. Such delays occur when consultants are not briefed during the induction programme, and informed of the drug formulary. This gap in communication resulted in the delay of the patient's treatment.

Advice: Casualty managers and/or casualty doctors must ensure the availability of medicines or implants before admitting any plan case to avoid any stressful situation.

Case study 2:

Sequence of events that led to the complete breakdown in administrative control

a. An ICU patient was admitted under a physician at 8am.

b. The physician came at 8.15am and wrote a referral to the cardiologist.

c. The cardiologist came at 8.45am and wrote a referral to the neurologist.

d. The Neurologist came at 8pm and recommended a CT scan of the brain.

e. CT was done at 8.05pm – almost twelve hours after the patient had arrived.

Who is at fault here?

Root-cause findings:

1. The protocols of the hospital/ICU were not followed.

2. Checklists and the SOPs were not followed.

[Note: The concerned doctors must see the patient in emergency/ICU at the earliest or at least within 45 minutes. In case the doctors do not come to see the patient, the next consultant doctor would have to be called after 45 minutes on the same day. This was not followed.]

It was a very rare case where the ward manager/sister in charge had not done their duties to inform the neurologist to come and see the patient. In such cases where the neurologists don't come to the ICU, the ICU manager and sister in charge should inform the medical superintendent, ICU doctors and administrator to take corrective measures. Thankfully, the patient recovered as the CT scan showed only a treatable problem, and the ICU doctor swiftly started the treatment as the neurologist recommended.

Action taken:

The management penalized the ward manager and the sister in charge with a deduction of a day's salary.

Case study 3:

Even the smallest things matter in hospital services. Once a patient came from out of town. The consultant had recommended three tests on him. Two tests were done in laboratories and for the last test, which was a non-invasive echocardiogram test, the doctors advised him to come with a report. He went to the non-invasive diagnostics department, where he was told to come the next day as already many patients were already waiting in a long queue.

The patient requested the OPD manager to get his test done on the same day as he had nowhere to stay in the town that night. However, the manager refused to help. When the administration received the information, they ensured all the tests were carried out swiftly. All reports came in the evening, the patient was seen by the doctor and the patient left happy and satisfied.

What went wrong?

1. The OPD manager did not take any initiative to prioritize the patient's tests.

2. Because of the OPD manager's failure to understand the patient's genuine problem, the patient had to reach out to higher officials, who ultimately helped him. Therefore, a case that should have been solved at the lower level ended up with higher management causing unnecessary stress.

Case study 4:

This was a unique problem. Once, a very anxious and concerned patient's attendant insisted upon one particular drug and even asked for more tests to be done on the patient. He also sought other doctors' opinions.

However, these requests were politely turned down. As a result, the patient attendant became agitated and started quarrelling.

This made the hospital administrator intervene.

He patiently listened to what the attendant had to say, coordinated with the relevant doctors to review the case. Still, the attendant was not satisfied. At that point, the treating consultant came and answered the attendant's queries about the treatment. In the meantime, the administrator quickly made plans B and C should the attendant still remain unconvinced.

There are other cases where the hospital administrator plays a key role.

For example, in some hospitals, once the patient's insurance (like in GIPSA cases) is denied, the hospital billing staff gives a revised bill, which is generally 15 to 18 per cent more than the TPA. Many times, it has been observed that the attendant insists on paying the TPA bill amount only. Such situations arise when patients' attendants are not briefed in advance of the frequently asked questions (FAQ) at the admission counter or by the casualty manager, ICU manager, ward manager.

In such situations, the administrator settles the bill taking all factors into account.

A medical superintendent or an administrative manager must teach their subordinate managers that the patient's interests are paramount. In other words, right at the time of the patient admission, the billing executive and the treating consultant must provide the attendant the full picture of the patient's treatment. This is important to ensure the attendant trusts the hospital fully and minimize the risk of patient-hospital conflict. A patient's satisfaction is key to the success of any hospital.

"The key to avoid patient-hospital conflict is to always give the full picture of the treatment and a fair estimate of the costs to the patient's side." – VBJ

Lesson 3

Small things matter

If the staff don't handle them properly, it may result in a huge loss to the hospital. Let us discuss why it is important to be very careful even while dealing with apparently small things with an imaginary case study of a fire incident.

Case study:

Let us first take one such imaginary incident from the maintenance department. One day, the hospital maintenance department's wielding staff wanted to work with a welding machine near the emergency gate. For this, they shifted the machine to the site.

But what do the fire-safety protocols say?

1. Safety parameters should be checked by a fire department officer before any welding work is done.

2. Fire department must give a green signal to carry out the welding work.

3. The supervisor of the maintenance department should be present on the site where any welding work is being carried out.

The maintenance staff thought that it was minor work that would hardly take five minutes and, hence, there was no point in calling the fire officer.

However, as soon as a maintenance worker started using the welding machine at the emergency area, fire sparks dropped to the ground, where there was already a great deal of generator oil due to leakage. This resulted in a major fire in the area.

Due to a stroke of luck, the fire officer arrived just in time and immediately cut off the electric connection, switched off the generator and then poured a shower of water from the sprinkler to contain the fire. If the fire had not been contained, it could have ended up with a loss of property and/or life. The casualty staff then announced "code red" and the patients were shifted to a safer area from the emergency department.

The root-cause findings of why this happened are:

1. Mandatory safety protocols were not followed resulting in negligence.

2. The safety inspection by the fire officer was not conducted and no permission was given by the fire department.

3. The generator was running and no one took any initiative to switch off the generator until the welding procedure was over, nor did anyone notice the oil leakage on the floor.

Conclusion:

The maintenance department was overconfident and bypassed the system while totally ignoring the protocols.

Advice: Any type of work, no matter how small or large, should not be taken lightly. Mock drills should be conducted regularly to keep the staff on their toes. The non-medical administrator/medical superintendent must ensure that safety protocols during hazardous work are always followed.

Recommendations:

1. A fire-detection system must be installed and properly maintained so that immediate action could be taken in case of a fire.

2. Safety protocols should be kept in mind always. For example, keeping a sufficient quantity of water, sand, and fire extinguisher at vulnerable places.

3. Special precaution should be taken where inflammables, like petrol and diesel, are kept.

4. Special safety measures must be taken for keeping stacks of paper in the record room.

5. Regular checks on devices that run on electricity, like fans, transformers, electrical boards, etc, and there should be ample ventilation as per protocol.

6. Regular renewal of annual maintenance contracts of all equipment installed to ensure their 24/7 serviceability.

7. Energy-saving audits to estimate the cost effectiveness of all expenditure incurred.

8. Most important rule for fire safety is known by its abbreviation – RACR. It stands for:

   a. **R**ace: Race to the spot of the incident.

   b. **A**larm: Sound the alarm for code red or call the fire brigade if the staff cannot contain the fire.

   c. **C**ontain. Try to combat and contain the fire.

   d. **R**escue. Rescue people and move them to safer places.

Advice: Hospital planners and academics should educate hospital management graduates about fire safety, code red, mock drills, prevention of fire techniques. This is to ensure that whenever such a situation arises, the hospital administrator does not panic and faces the situation calmly.

Important point to remember:

We can't blame the lower staff for all mistakes. It is the collective responsibility of the head of all departments who supervise the lower staff's work. If department heads are careless, they can bring more harm to the hospital. Therefore, the administrator must be tough. He should not allow too much friendliness between staff members. This may result in the dilution of the gravity of a colleague's mistake or may result in the failure to pinpoint the blame on a colleague.

"The administrator should be task-oriented and assign a time frame for each task to his subordinate, monitor them closely by giving his or her best advice and get the work done efficiently from the team."
– VBJ

Lesson 3A

Home collection of samples

Often, the hospital sends laboratory technicians to collect blood, urine, and other samples from people's homes. It is a very specialized task. The hospital must send only trained staff for this. Otherwise, it may result in unnecessary issues.

Let us discuss this with an imaginary case study to highlight this.

Case study:

Once, a person requested the hospital to collect his blood sample from his home as he was called to his office during the time he was supposed to visit the hospital to give his blood sample for testing. The hospital sent a technician to collect the sample along with the person's phone number. When the technician contacted the person, the person requested the technician to collect his sample from the Metro station, from where he would catch the train to his office.

The technician was a novice who had joined the hospital only recently. He accepted the request and went to the area near the Metro station where the person asked him to meet. Without consulting his superior on this matter, he started taking blood samples from the person in full public view. A police officer watching them from a distance came near and asked what was going on. Then people started gathering around them and soon rumours, like "drug peddlers are operating openly", started to float around. Sensing trouble, the officer took both of them to the police station for interrogation. Meanwhile the lab technician called his senior who called the security officer and administrator to sort out the issue.

The administrator and the chief security officer went to the police station, apologized for the sad incident and informed the police that the technician was a hospital staffer and there was no foul play. Thankfully, the matter ended there and both the technician and the person were freed.

The administrator briefed the head of the laboratory & diagnostics department on the incident and instructed him to carry out corrective measures so that such a situation doesn't arise in the future.

Root-cause findings:

1. This mistake happened due to the ignorance of the laboratory technician.
2. The head of the laboratory & diagnostics department should have briefed him about the dos and don'ts or, at least, should have asked the technician's seniors to do the same.
3. The department sent a novice for home collection of samples, which is the work of those technicians who are fully acquainted with the job.

Guideline for laboratory technicians:

No laboratory technician from the laboratory & diagnostics' home collection section is authorized to take samples from public places, like parks, hotel lobbies, markets, transport stations, etc. They are only authorized to do so at the address registered with the home collection section.

Word of caution:

A collecting technician may face situations that may cause delay in collecting samples from homes, like his vehicle breaking down, a mishap or an accident, etc. This causes great stress and anxiety in the person whose samples are to be collected. Therefore, if there is an appointment for home collection, the home collection section's coordinator must remain in touch with the technician. The coordinator should always have a Plan B ready, like a backup technician on standby, whenever such a situation arises.

Lesson 3B

Maintenance department issues

The maintenance department is a very important department in a hospital. All hospital departments depend upon its efficient handling of everything – from electricity to infrastructure. Every department in the hospital must have serviceability clearance from the maintenance department. Even small issues, if not handled professionally, can lead to accidents and unnecessary stress for the administrator and management. Finally, if necessary, the administrator must settle the issue.

Let us take two imaginary incidents as case studies.

Incident 1:

Once a female patient was admitted in a private room. She decided to work on her laptop. She put two pillows on her back for support on the reclining bed, which are common in most hospitals, and adjusted the curve of the bed in such a way that she was comfortable. Suddenly, the lever that curves or straightens the bed detached and the part of the bed that was curved towards her back supporting her crashed. The patient fell on her back without warning and injured her head. Fortunately, the two pillows that she had tucked between the bed and her back minimized the impact and the injury was mild.

She reported the matter to the administrator. A probe found that the bed was repaired 15 days before the incident because a similar thing had happened. However, the maintenance department didn't take the issue seriously and fixed it by just putting the faulty lever in its earlier place.

The ward manager intelligently shifted the patient to the next bed, the malfunctioning bed was replaced and sent for condemnation by the administrator. The ward manager handled the whole incident calmly and did not show any sign of nervousness. At one time, the patient's husband was furious and threatened to share the photos of the bed on social media. The administrator and ward manager apologized for such an unfortunate incident and assured him that this would not happen again.

The administrator also instructed the maintenance staff to be proactive in such cases, so that they are not repeated.

Incident 2:

A very serious patient came to the emergency department, and the doctor announced code blue within two to three minutes. The ICU team arrived to save the life of the patient and instructed the casualty doctor to shift the patient to the cardiac ICU at the earliest, as the patient had just suffered a heart attack. The casualty manager coordinated with all the people involved in the case, arranged a green corridor to shift the patient to the cardiac ICU. The patient was given cardiopulmonary resuscitation (CPR) as his blood pressure had dropped drastically.

Everything was going as per protocol until the patient was moved to the lift area.

Just as the patient was brought to the lift to change floors, the electricity went off. The operator immediately informed the maintenance department and asked it to start the generator. Luckily, this was promptly done and the lift started working within a couple of minutes. The patient was able to be shifted to the cardiac ICU just in time.

Observation:

The casualty manager had coordinated with almost everyone, but did not tell the lift operator or the maintenance office to keep everything in generator mode. The casualty manager handled the situation in such a way that their attendant did not know if there was an electricity outage. While there was no nervousness shown by any staff, they were also not aware of the true reason behind the delay in taking the patient to the ICU. If not for the quick-thinking lift operator, this sensitive issue could have become a major problem.

Advices:

a. *Before shifting any patient, ensure a checklist of rooms, facilities, other things that would be needed during the transit.*

b. *Never go by "yes, sir" or "all well, sir" verbally. Always make sure the checklist is ticked correctly.*

c. *Whenever any serious "code blue" patient is being shifted using the lift, the administrator must inform everyone concerned, including the maintenance department, to keep lift on generator mode for the safe passage of the patient.*

Lesson 3C

Billing complaints

Most of the administrators in private hospitals almost always face billing complaints in one form or another. The hospital administrator should always take a progressive and 360° approach to settle such cases.

Let us discuss two imaginary incidents to highlight the importance of deft handling of such cases.

Incident 1:

Once, a patient's final bill for a cataract surgery was ₹55,000. However, the patient's attendant wanted a discount from the billing HOD, which was refused. The attendant of the patient then asked for a component-wise breakdown of the bill. It was given to the attendant as below:

	Component	Bill (in ₹)
1	Day care	1,500
2	Nursing care	300
3	Eye surgeon charges	22,000
4	OT charges	12,400
5	OT consumables	400
6	External medicine	800
7	Lens	17,000
Total		**55,000**

The patient's attendant then raised two questions – one original and one a follow-up query. He first asked:

"If the OT consumables cost just ₹400 and the external medicines ₹800, then why an extra ₹12,400 was charged?" *[Note: The attendant's query was absolutely legitimate.]*

The HOD of the billing department thus replied:

"The surgeon's fee was ₹22,400. According to the hospital's billing policy, the OT charges are 55 per cent of the surgeon fees. Therefore, the hospital charged the amount of ₹12,400."

Then the patient's attendant then followed this up with his second query:

"Why the OT charges were 55 per cent of the surgeon's fee, why not 25 per cent or 10 per cent?"

The billing HOD stuck to his previous point in answering the second question. He said:

"It was the billing policy of the hospital."

The patient's attendant was not convinced and complained to the chief administrator, asking him to examine the breakup of the bill and consider his request for some discount. The chief administrator assured him that he would consider his grievance earnestly. The chief administrator met the medical superintendent and together, they helped the patient by giving him a discount on the bill. The patient paid the bill and left satisfied.

The chief administrator in a hospital is always there to help patients in need, especially to those who come in distress and agony.

Other issues which can be the bone of contention between a patient and the hospital are: differences in bills, TPA package, ward charges, ICU charges, exclusion of non-consumable in TPAs, etc.

The logic hospitals give for the difference in billing are often the following:

a. Sometimes, the cost of medicines, consumables and treatment exceeds the amount in the package.

b. Cost of implants, like stents, are more than the price cap panel companies fix.

*[**Note:** Generally no private hospital wants to bear losses due to the differential amount between expenses incurred versus the amount of money fixed by the package.]*

Sometimes, there is a difference between the actual bill and the amount fixed in the patients' treatment package. Sometimes it takes a full day to explain such cases. In some cases, the management takes into account several factors to settle bill disputes.

The chief administrator always gives clear instructions to all managers to keep a watch on expenses and treatment, as well as to inform the patients and/or their attendants. For example, if the expenses exceed the amount in the treatment package, like the cost of an implant is more than what is capped in the package, the patients and/or their attendants must be informed before the procedure/surgery to avoid disputes when the final bill is made.

Lesson 4

Media and healthcare sector

A new phenomenon in the healthcare sector is the interference of traditional mainstream media, like print or electronic media, and social media, like Facebook, Twitter, YouTube, WhatsApp, etc. This has changed the people's mindset and behaviour. Earlier print and electronic media gave information about good research or the achievements of a doctor to the general public and they are still doing it. Additionally, they make the public aware of issues, like pollution, disease outbreaks, health and lifestyle issues, etc.

However, these days, a patient's problems and/or their attendant's grievances are quickly latched on to and sensationalized by both the mainstream media and social media users. This new trend has brought new concerns for the healthcare sector, especially the hospitals.

At times, mainstream and social media disseminated information that were fake or one-sided or were half-truths to sensationalize them in order to grab more eyeballs and traction from social media users. Sometimes, major players with vested interests encourage such reporting or spreading of such information.

Apart from these, patients and/or their attendants take to social media if their grievances are not addressed immediately and according to their demands. In some cases, especially if a patient dies, the attendant calls reporters, who then start inquiring about the patient's treatment.

Some of the questions (FAQs) that reporters may ask in such events are:

a. Name of the patient.

b. Date of admission.

c. About the patient's prognosis and the treatment given.

d. Inquiring about allegations by a patient attendant, such as medical negligence during treatment, extra charges in bill, doctors and diagnostic reports not made available on time, not given correct/complete information, etc.

e.   Other miscellaneous questions.

Real challenge for an administrator

The hospital administrator must retain composure and not overreact when such situations arise. If a patient's attendant calls the media, the administrator should meet the attendant and at the same time arrange for a meeting between the attendant and the treating doctors, medical superintendent and representatives of higher management, where everything is explained to address the attendant's grievances or doubts.

If needed, the administrator should release a statement for the media to counter the grieving attendant's allegation. In rare cases, a hospital might be required to send official documents to the district or city magistrate or the local police station house officer about the real status of the patient.

Sometimes, the hospital's security stops media persons from entering the hospital or particular areas like the ICU or ward to meet the grieving attendant who called them. This often results in arguments and unnecessary stress for the administrator.

It should be noted that mainstream media and social media are nobody's friends, nor anybody's enemy. As the situation develops, mainstream media and social media react accordingly. One piece of wrong information may lead to another, which may lead to the spread of misinformation. Then it becomes a problem for the hospital. The hospital's management stands united whenever such a situation arises and deals with all problems fairly. Always try for a solution to move forward in the interests of both the patients and the hospital.

It has also been observed that sometimes human rights activists, police officials, government health officials and even district or city magistrates start inquiring about cases that the media carried. In worst cases, some patients' attendants/relatives may themselves go to the police or a court to lodge their complaint, if they remain dissatisfied with the explanations the hospitals gave them. To handle such cases, the hospital employs legal advisers to counter patients' or their attendants' allegations. However, it is of paramount importance that the management must keep all possible options open to arrive at an amicable settlement with the patients or their attendants.

Generally the hospital administrator interacts with media on two issues:

1. **For an event:** When hospital authorities send them invitations for coverage on events, such as an inauguration of a new treatment facility, induction of new technology in treatment, etc, and during news conferences, public lectures, etc.

2. **During an incident:** The media is called by the grieving patient or patient's attendant.

Important:

Based on my experience as an administrator, there is no fixed formula for handling media. Before talking to the media, the medical superintendent and/or the treating consultant and/or the hospital's spokesperson and/or a representative of the hospital's higher management do all the homework and crosscheck everything.

Other side of the story:

Most mainstream media organizations are still doing a great job for the healthcare sector by highlighting the sector's achievements, like research by a pharmaceutical company or a good job done by a hospital. Such things always get prime space in the media.

The hospital's marketing team, who are instrumental in building the branding of the hospital, interact with the media most of the time. They are the ones who mostly arrange for news conferences in and outside the hospital. Journalists have easy access to the medical superintendent and the hospital administrator. If they need to meet higher authorities, their meetings are generally arranged.

Social media helps in building the brand of a hospital and the hospital's marketing department usually employs people who are experts in handling social media.

Another new trend that may become problematic for the hospital:

These days, many patients raise funds through apps developed for the purpose or via social media campaigns. These apps and campaigns require the patient's case summary, an estimate of treatment charges, etc. Patients or their attendants generally don't take the hospital's permission to share such private and often sensitive information on the app or to the social media campaigners. This may become problematic for the hospital in case something goes wrong.

Let us discuss such an imaginary incident to highlight the issue.

Incident:

Once, a very sick newborn was put on the ventilator. The hospital gave the baby's parents an estimate of ₹3 lakh for keeping the baby in the neonatal ICU for 15 days. Since they didn't have the money, they opted to go for a fundraiser through an app for this purpose.

As the baby's parents were not tech savvy, they took the help of a person who said he could help them. Apparently, the person was a con man. He put an extra zero in the sum making the estimate ₹30 lakh, doctored the case summary and uploaded it on the app for approval of the fundraising campaign. The organization behind the app naturally called the hospital to authenticate the case as a large amount of money was involved. The administrator was informed, who then called the baby's parents and asked for the details. This led to the identification of the person who tried to swindle them and the matter was reported to the authorities.

Thought for curriculum planners:

Media management, including mainstream media, social media, and digital media marketing must be included in the hospital management curriculum. It must include lessons on the role and impact of media on hospitals in today's scenario. If this is taught, newcomers will be vigilant and will not be blindsided whenever a tricky or a difficult situation presents itself unexpectedly. This will also enable these non-medicos to become effective spokespersons or brand managers of a hospital.

Lesson 4A

Importance of keeping focus on work

Administrative problems are generally manageable in most cases. One of my own observations as an administrator is that most of the problems in hospitals are usually self-created due to human error, that is, the staff not taking their job seriously or working without focus. Sometimes, heavy footfall in the hospital or extra workload causes a staffer to make mistakes, like forgetting to follow the standard operating procedure or not going thoroughly through a checklist.

People come to hospitals due to necessity and not for any sightseeing or entertainment. It is a sensitive and emotional place. The staff must show empathy, be polite and courteous and always concentrate 100 per cent on their work. They must never pass on the responsibility from one person to another carelessly.

Let us take three imaginary case studies to stress on the importance of focus during work.

Incident 1:

Once, a patient's attendant complained that the plate on which food was served to the patient had a rusted spoon and yellowish tissue paper. He asked for an explanation from the kitchen manager, who apologized and changed the plate's spoon and tissue paper. The patient attendant put the rusted spoon and tissue paper in a small bag. On the next day, he met the chief administrator and showed him the spoon and the tissue paper. On inquiry, his complaint was found to be correct, the chief administrator apologized to him and assured him that such an incident would not happen in future.

The administrator, showing empathy, then inquired about the patient's health. Thankfully, the patient, who was the attendant's mother, was stable and about to be discharged. The chief administrator gave a discount on the billed amount and the patient and their attendant left happy and satisfied.

The chief administrator then called a meeting with the dietician/kitchen manager and advised him/her to be more careful while serving food. All the food served must be as per the hospital's policy and regular checks should be carried out to prevent even small issues.

Incident 2:

Once a patient received a small and overripe banana as a part of his meal. Her son, who was also her attendant, called the ward manager, who in turn called the chief administrator and the dietician/kitchen manager. The attendant showed the banana to them. The chief administrator advised the dietician/kitchen manager to ensure that only fresh and edible fruits are served to patients. The chief administrator, showing empathy and gratitude, then inquired about the health of the attendant's mother and wished her a speedy recovery.

Incident 3:

A patient was admitted to the cardiac care unit (CCU). He had a heart attack and urgently required a primary angioplasty. However, the patient's attendant didn't have the money to pay for it. The manager asked his superiors for permission to carry out the treatment anyway, and was allowed to do so immediately.

The angioplasty was immediately carried out and the ward manager gave the patient a general ward package. The next day, a newly appointed ward manager came to CCU and found zero deposit in a case file that gave the patient a double-bed package, which was higher than the earlier one. The patient's attendant met the chief administrator and showed him both the estimates.

The chief administrator studied the case and assured the attendant that in their case, the general ward package was applicable. In the evening, the patient's condition worsened and he expired. The bill was made via a general ward package as instructed by the chief administrator. The attendant came and met the chief administrator to request some discount as the patient expired. The request was accepted and the bill was further discounted.

The next day, the chief administrator called both the managers and told them not to repeat this mistake and follow the hospital guidelines:

1. Managers must be briefed on the estimate of the bill at the time of handing over the charge by other managers and copies of the estimates must be kept in the case file of the patient to avoid any misunderstanding.

2. There should be proper explanations in case of any changes in treatment or packages, like upgrading from general ward to double bed or double bed to single private room, etc, that may affect the final bill substantially. This goes a long way to retain patients and their attendants' trust in the hospital system.

"'Difficult' doesn't mean 'impossible'. It means you have to work hard to solve problems with confidence and commitment." – VBJ

Lesson 4B

Patient dissatisfaction, psychology of patient and attendants

Dissatisfaction among patients is a very sensitive issue. It is very difficult to pinpoint at what stage a patient and/or a patient's attendant become(s) dissatisfied in the hospital during the course of the patient's treatment and becomes agitated and even aggressive.

The hospital always works to save the life of a patient by trying to give them the best-possible treatment, and with all the resources it has. Also, the hospital always tries to give its frank and honest opinion regarding prognosis, even if it is a serious or a terminal condition. Apart from this, if deemed necessary, a hospital may refer a patient to a better equipped hospital of their choice for better treatment. Also, in some cases, like when an organ transplantation is required, and the hospital is not equipped to do such operations, it may refer the patient to a hospital where such facilities are available.

Having said so, based upon my experiences as a hospital administrator, I have found the following reasons to be the most common to trigger patient dissatisfaction:

1. Long stay in hospital.

2. Patients and attendants want everything to be done as they want.

3. They want their cases to be handled on a priority basis, seek favours in consultation, get laboratory & diagnostics reports at the earliest, getting special attention beyond the doctor's scope during treatment, etc.

4. TPA denial/billing disputes.

5. In rare cases, when a young patient passes away during the course of treatment.

6. Alleged negligence by medical/non-medical staff.

7. When the sole breadwinner in the family is admitted.

8. When a large number of local people are admitted at the same time.

9. Attendants' or relatives' fear of loss, stress, tension, short temper and anxiety.

10. Sudden deterioration of a patient's condition.

11. Other reasons.

Sometimes, a patient and/or the patient's attendant might suddenly get dissatisfied and become hyper aggressive at any stage during the course of the patient's treatment. In such situations, "code violet" is declared, and security and the administrator try to solve the issue. However, in some cases, the grievances of the patient's relatives become a threat to law and order. In such a scenario, the administrator consults the management and then calls the police to safeguard the hospital and ensure no harm is done to either the staff or other patients and their attendants. Nonetheless, the first objective remains to resolve the issue amicably.

All hospitals treat their patients and interact with their attendants with dignity, respect and compassion. However, during the course of treatment, if a patient feels dissatisfied, then the administrator meets the patient and/or the patient's attendant and tries to help by:

1. Reviewing the case with the treating doctors.

2. Review the case with another doctor for a second opinion.

3. Initiate a meeting of the ethical committee comprising the treating doctors, medical superintendent and representative of the senior management to resolve the issue.

4. Hospitals prepare a case summary with all details and hand it over to the patient's side for a second opinion from another hospital, if they so want, and respect their decision for a referral/LAMA/DOR.

Thoughts for curriculum planners:

1. The hospital management graduate must be educated on human psychological behaviour in detail, especially the psychology of patients and their attendants. Having knowledge of the same will help an administrator handle such situations with ease.

2. Hospital management graduates must also be educated about the psychology of staff (both medical and non-medical). It must focus on

how to discharge their duties in a professional way so that there are no mistakes from the hospital's end and the patient leaves the hospital satisfied.

"Many times, patients and/or their kin compliment the hospital and its staff for their excellent service. This shouldn't make the staff complacent, which may lead to serious lapses in service. Hence, always follow SOPs and protocols in place." – VBJ

Lesson 4C

Administrative challenges for VVIP/VIP/general patients

Based on the person's status in society, the following types of people come to a hospital for treatment:

1. Patients from the general public.

2. VVIP or VIP patients.

3. Convicts, arrested suspects in police custody who need treatment.

Patients from the general public:

Most of the members of the general public abide by the law of the land, meet the doctors waiting for their turn and follow the hospital's protocols. The administrator and security in charge just perform a supervisory role.

That said, the hospital administrator must give priority to members of the general public who are: handicapped, mentally challenged, psychiatric patients, senior citizens and the bedridden. And above all, prioritize those patients who require urgent treatment and are not in a position to wait. The administrator must show empathy and help to all of them.

In the psychiatry OPD, the administrator must depute a security staff to keep an eye on the activities of the psychiatric patients. Sometimes, psychiatric patients can become violent and can harm anyone indiscriminately. Therefore, it calls for security staff in the area to remain alert so that they can manage the situation and doctors can provide immediate treatment to calm the patient without violating the system.

VVIP and VIP patients:

VIPs come to hospitals for mainly two purposes. They are:

1. For medical tests, consultation and treatment.

2. To meet their family members, friends, associates who are admitted in the hospital.

In both cases, the hospital authorities, the security in charge and the administration department should remain on high alert and make all the arrangements from the moment the VIP enters the hospital.

The entire route should be managed by the administrator with the help of security in order to prove a hassle free arrangement without disturbing the system and harassment to other patients already in the hospital.

Sometimes, the VIP's assistant or his official, who accompany the VIP, sends messages to the media announcing the VIP's arrival at the hospital. As a result, media persons come to the hospital to interview the VIP and/or report on the visit. In such situations, the administrator and the hospital's security in charge face difficulty in handling the journalists as well as the crowd, which generally gathers inside the hospital. If the VIP wants to talk to the media then the administrator should provide a suitable place for an interview.

Regarding treatment for a VIP, the administrator should help in everything: consultations, tests, procedures, even admissions to make them comfortable.

The VIP's entire route within the hospital is managed by the administrator with the help of the security in charge without disturbing the systems.

The administrator and security chief should also request the VIP's bodyguards to sit in the designated area to avoid crowding. However, in some cases, the bodyguards don't listen and insist on being in close proximity to the VIP throughout their stay in the hospital. If the police or the paramilitary officers are in the VIP's security detail, the administrator goes by their preference.

If a VIP is visiting a local area, the police and local intelligence official comes with a dog squad, bomb disposal squad, other gadgets and the fire brigade remains in and around the hospital in case of an emergency in which the hospital's services are needed.

On such occasions, the hospital administrator helps in arranging a "safe house" for the VIP with all emergency medicines and puts doctors on standby. The hospital authorities, the hospital administrator, the hospital security in charge stay on high alert and make all the arrangements.

After the VIP leaves the hospital, the administrator announces the departure to all concerned staff so that they may return to their work.

The administrator must have experience and exposure in handling VIP visits to hospitals. He should be able to instruct his staff in a code language, which can be developed in consultation with various departments.

[Note: It should be mentioned that hospital management doesn't discriminate on the basis of caste, creed, religion and social status of patients. All are equal in the eyes of the hospital. However, to avoid certain issues, all major hospitals have no choice but to distinguish between a VIP and a member of the general public, and give the VIPs special attention and favours.]

Patients who are convicts or suspects in police custody:

Police sometimes bring convicts and suspects in their custody to a hospital for treatment if they fall sick or have a sustained injury while in custody or during their arrest or during an encounter to arrest them. Here too, the administrator and the security in charge arrange everything for the patient. The hospital security is put on high alert at entry and exit points to avoid any unpleasant situations, like an escape attempt by the patient or an attempt by the patient's gang members to rescue him from law enforcement's custody.

Things to remember:

Every hospital has a "visitors policy". However, in some countries, like in India, most people live in closely-knit families and are well connected with their extended families, friends and relatives. During the hospitalization of a friend, relative or an associate, it is part of the Indian culture to visit them to know about the status of the patient's or just to cheer and motivate the patient. If a patient is from a rural background, even more people come to see the patient. This makes handling the visitors difficult for the administration and security.

Advice: Always refrain from using harsh words on visitors.

"Visitors are the hospital's brand ambassadors. Their word-of-mouth publicity is better than any other medium. Therefore, administrators and security managers should follow a balanced, flexible and diplomatic approach when handling visitors." – VBJ

Lesson 5

Handling everyday problems in the ICU and ward

The ICU and the ward of a hospital throw up routine challenges and have routine problems to fix. Some of the routine problems medical superintendents and chief administrators face during their rounds in the ICU and wards are as follows:

1. On-duty ICU/ward staff are found asleep at night.

2. Doctors don't see the patient at night despite repeated reminders.

3. Doctors write a referral in the evening, but the referral consultant doesn't see the patient at night and the patient expires.

4. In some cases, the staff forget to get the attendant's signature on the patient's prognosis before the patient expires.

5. The ICU staff fail to inform the consultant doctor of a patient's expiry.

6. In rare cases, ward boys or the housekeeping staff use the same gloves while handling more than one patient.

7. Sometimes nurses don't know the local language and find it difficult to communicate.

8. In rare cases, pharmacies deliver wrong medicines.

9. In certain cases, where the condition of the patient is serious or the patient can't help himself or is immobile, problems arise when making the patient take medicines or food.

10. Make arrangements for immediate surgery.

11. Patient's condition suddenly worsens and they expire despite doctors giving a positive outlook on the patient's recovery.

In such cases the role of the medical superintendent, chief administrator, and all those who are dealing with patient care become very tough.

Suggestion:

Try to pacify the attendant and not allow politics or arguments or differences to cause the situation to slip out of control. The hospital administrator must listen to both the hospital's side and the patient's side. Sometimes one-sided stories may result in an unsavoury escalation of the issue. However, when the administrator listens carefully to both sides, they can arrive at a peaceful solution.

If a need arises, the administrator should brief the higher management regarding an issue and try to settle it as soon as possible and move forward.

Things to remember:

Never lose composure. Be calm and help to create a healthy environment where everyone has mutual respect for each other. People expect good services from a private hospital such as:

a. Safety.

b. Good hygienic practices.

c. Good nursing care.

d. High-end OT, laboratory & diagnostic, emergency services.

e. Prompt reliable treatment by the senior doctors.

f. ICLS ambulances.

g. Good ambience and comfort.

A satisfied patient and/or the patient's attendant will tell his friends and relatives the good things about the hospital. However, an unsatisfied patient and/or the patient's attendant will tell many more people the bad things about the hospital. The job of the administrator is to keep in mind the image and interests of the hospital and show empathy while dealing with the patients and/or their attendants.

It is important for hospital administrators to keep in mind that they are dealing with lives and not products. The importance of saving a patient's life is paramount and does not require a lengthy discussion to elaborate on this. The earlier you understand the problems, the faster you find the solutions.

Handling death cases

Death is a very emotional issue and the administrator must be extra cautious in dealing with death cases. Sometimes, issues arise while settling bills after a patient dies during the course of treatment. All private hospitals handle this with compassion and an all-round approach. However, in rare cases, there may be a problem where a patient's relatives start quarrelling while settling bills and make the environment tense. The administrator should always try for a peaceful settlement and move forward.

TPA settlement is another issue that gets complicated when a patient dies. In most of these cases, the patients' attendants always want to leave early with the body, but time taken for the TPA clearance takes time.

In certain cases, a patient who is admitted for showing a symptom for an ailment and whose treatment is covered by TPA is diagnosed with a different ailment that is not covered by it. For example, a patient admitted for chest pain gets a report on further investigation that the pain was a result of stones in the gallbladder, for which there was no TPA cover, instead of a cardiac ailment, which had TPA cover. Such situations can become problematic for the ward, ICU or the hospital administrator.

Medico-legal cases (MLC) are always troublesome in death cases. The police handle most of the aspects of an MLC with the help of administration and the housekeeping department staff, including shifting the corpse from the hospital to the postmortem facility.

Now, let us discuss such a case.

Case:

In a medicolegal case, a patient expired at 4.47am. When the patient's attendant came to take the dead body, the hospital staff informed him that as it was an MLC, the police will allow the handing over of the body only after the postmortem formalities are completed.

The dead patient's attendant waited until 9am, but no policeman came. The attendant inquired what was going on at the reception. The administration also got the message and followed it up. He was shocked to learn that the death memo had not been sent to the police station. The administrator then took everything in his hands and contacted the police and requested them to come urgently for completing the postmortem formalities. Within half an hour, a police officer came and started all the formalities and the patient's dead body was shifted to the postmortem house by 10.30am.

Root-cause analysis:

The root of the problem lies in the question: **Why was the death memo not sent on time?**

It was found that the night manager was on leave and the new manager who was working didn't know the procedures of sending a death memo to the police station. Only when the administrator came to know about it and took matters into his hands, things started moving. The administrator instructed the night manager that in such cases, he or other senior officers of the hospital should be contacted immediately so that such incidents can be avoided in future.

Advice: *During the induction program, everyone should be briefed on the duties of the staff. So that if a real situation arises, people will know what to do and not leave it all to others.*

Sometimes, in the cases where patients die, their attendants may claim that extra charges were added to the bill or seek a discount even after the billing in charge breaks down the bill and explains everything in detail. In such cases, the chief administrator or the medical superintendent should show compassion. He/she should also have all the documents from the dead patient's case file to confidently try to convince the attendant that the doctors tried their best to save the patient. This is to ensure that their faith on the hospital remains strong.

In cases where people from deceased patients' side confront the hospital and make the environment tense, the entire hospital management should show unity, compassion and think from all the angles to settle the issue amicably.

The administrator's job is not a simple one. The hospital management has to accept that to run the hospital smoothly, swift solutions and actions by the administrator are needed. A simple case, if not handled properly, can quickly escalate into a crisis.

"Each and every problem has a solution. Refresh, restart, refocus, review as many times you can. Don't quit until the problem is solved either by you or by others or by both others and you." – VBJ

Lesson 5A

Challenges during Covid-19 pandemic

The responsibility of hospital administrators increased manyfold during the lockdown and afterwards due to the Covid-19 pandemic in 2020. Higher pressure, longer working hours, emotional stress, etc, was on an unprecedented scale among hospital workers. It also brought new and unforeseen challenges to keep the hospitals' business running and managing it well.

Wave I

When the phase one, which we refer to as "Wave I", of the pandemic hit the country, the Union government imposed a very strict lockdown at a very short notice bringing the country to a grinding halt. Then, new decisions, protocols and guidelines were implemented.

The biggest challenge was to implement the new decisions according to the protocol of the Union home ministry, state government and the Indian Council of Medical Research during the first wave of the pandemic. The orders from these organizations were constantly evolving, which kept the hospital management on their toes 24/7. This was happening even as hospital staff struggled to cope with the consequences of self-quarantine, Covid-19 treatment, Covid-19 hotspots (which were categorized as green zones and red zones), complete lockdowns.

Hospitals had to make arrangements for a flu corner to screen all patients and their attendants at the entry point and the protocols made by the in-house pathology department had to be implemented by the administrator at all the departments. There was one rule above all: **"No Mask, No Entry."**

The hospital's security became crucial to safeguard the well-being of the patients, their attendants and other visitors. Security guards were deployed at every level of the hospital to ensure:

a. They washed their hands with soap.

b. Go to the flu corner to get their temperature checked with a non-contact thermometer (gun thermometer).

They were also tasked to ask every new patient, their attendant and visitors to go to the flu corners where doctors and other staff asked them questions on:

1. Their native town/village.
2. The area they live in and whether it was a hotspot or not.
3. Their travelling history, like if they had been abroad recently.
4. If they had Covid-19 symptoms, like fever, cold and cough, etc. If the answer was positive, the duration of the symptoms.

Only after going through the Covid-screening process, patients, their attendants and visitors are allowed to enter the hospital.

The hospital management had also created infrastructure to protect its staff, patients and their attendants from Covid-19. New rules were made for attendants, like allowing only one attendant for a patient who is admitted in the ward or ICU and banning attendants to stay in the waiting area. If a treating doctor wanted to talk to a patient's attendant to explain the prognosis of the patient, the latter was allowed in the ICU. Furthermore, it was mandatory for patients' attendants to wear personal protective equipment (PPE) inside the ICU.

Such strict rules were not there before the outbreak of the pandemic.

Problems/issues Wave I brought for hospital administrators

There were several restrictions for even handling the smallest of issues, such as:

a. Small issues needed the administrator's intervention. For example: if a patient was unconscious/bedridden, the attendant couldn't leave until another person came to relieve him because the hospital barred new attendants to enter when one attendant was already inside the ward.

b. Once, a patient's attendant was already inside when the hospital authorities asked him to deposit money. He told the hospital that his brother was waiting outside and requested they allow him to pay as he was carrying a credit card. Here too, the administrator intervened and allowed his brother to come inside to make the payment.

c. Once, a Covid patient expired. The administrator ensured that his relatives would follow government rules to carry out his funeral. One of his relatives wanted to see the face of the deceased, whose body was packed in the hospital as per protocols. The administrator showed compassion and allowed the relative to see the deceased face, but only after taking all precautions.

Hospital administrators constantly motivated the hospital staff and ensured that all anti-Covid precautions were in place and protocols implemented.

Administrators had a difficult time dealing with issues, such as:

a. Staff quarantine.

b. Suspected Covid patients being asymptomatic.

c. Handling Covid cases.

d. Rostering staff.

e. Allaying infection fears among medicos and non-medicos.

f. Transporting staff.

g. Making arrangements for staff to stay in the hospital.

h. Covid testing for staff members who had Covid symptoms.

i. Radiologist staff and doctors who are exposed to Covid patients.

j. Transporting Covid patients or their dead bodies.

k. Handling waste and laundry of Covid patients.

l. Staff who were on leave couldn't return to work due to lockdown.

m. Staff living in hot spots couldn't report to work.

n. Daily-wage workers in hospitals not getting any work.

o. Maintaining separate entrances and lifts for Covid patients.

The abovementioned problems were just the tip of the iceberg. In reality, the problems and issues the pandemic brought for hospitals were endless.

The government also designated some hospitals to treat only Covid-19 patients. In such hospitals, they categorized the patients into three following categories as per their condition:

I. **L1**, where they were provided with beds with oxygen.
II. **L2**, where they were admitted to the ICU with no ventilator support.
III. **L3**, where they were admitted to the ICU with ventilator support.

The rates also fixed for treatment of the patients in the above categories.

Observations:

1. When a patient undergoing treatment in a non-Covid hospital is detected with Covid-19 infection, the hospital management advised the patient to get admitted in a Covid hospital. However, it has been observed that in many cases, getting a bed in a Covid-19 hospital was very difficult during the peak of the pandemic.
2. Seeing the Covid-19 patients' difficulty in getting beds, the local administration instructed the Covid hospitals to display the number of bed occupancy and vacant beds for each category (L1, L2, and L3).

Dealing with price hike of services

Case study:

The Covid pandemic increased the demand for ambulance and hearse services many times. This also opened up a window for unfair profiteering for some ambulance and hearse service providers, to whom most hospitals outsource the job. For example, normally, hiring a hearse from Noida to Ghazipur cremation ground normally costs ₹880 for 8 kilometres, but with expired Covid patients, these ambulance and hearse operators started charging as much as ₹4,500 to ₹5,000. In one such case, a hospital administrator got to know about it and probed the matter. The ambulance provider said they were charging higher for Covid patients or their dead bodies as they had to arrange for PPE kits for drivers and their helpers. In addition to this, they had to compensate the drivers for having to wait for a long time due to long queues at the cremation grounds, due to a surge in deaths.

Upon hearing this, the administrator cancelled the contract of the ambulance and hearse services provider and allowed the hospital's driver to transport corpses to the cremation ground by just giving him a PPE kit and ₹880.

It should also be noted that life-saving medicines were in short supply during the pandemic, which created panic among the general public.

Even ambulance services with life-supporting equipment were outsourced to agencies, who were charging ₹7,000 to ₹10,000 for 20km for transporting Covid patients, whereas the normal charges are ₹4,000 to ₹5,000.

Even for PPE kits, hospitals were charging ₹800 to ₹1,000 approximately and standalone shops were selling different versions of PPE kits for as low as ₹550 approximately. Explaining to the patients and/or their attendants about different PPE kits was another challenge to the hospital administration.

In the early days of the pandemic, the government capped the price for Covid testing to ₹4,500. However, when the steep rate triggered an outrage among the public, the price was reduced to ₹2,400 and then to ₹1,600. By December, it was further reduced and the price came down to just ₹700. This was a relief to the general public. Also, the new policy meant that it was now only mandatory for patients requiring a surgery/procedure to have a negative Covid RT-PCR test report.

Transporting a deceased from one state to another

Case study

Once, a very emotional incident happened when a patient arrived dead at the hospital. The attendant was new to Noida, where he came for a family visit but was stuck in the city due to the lockdown. The attendant wished to take the patient's body to Kerala for the last rites. However, this could have been possible only after completing the following formalities:

1. Getting the death memo from the hospital to the police station, along with the death certificate.

2. Postmortem report.

3. Covid test report.

4. No-objection certificate from the local police.

5. Embalming of the body for air transportation.

The administrator arranged everything from the death certificate to the death memo to ease the attendant's suffering and helped them take the body back to Kerala. The attendant was extremely grateful for the help.

Showing compassion to staff

Once, the bicycle of a ward boy was stolen from outside the hospital, where it was parked despite a clear sign saying "parking at owner's risk". The ward boy lodged a complaint in the hospital as well as the police station and requested the hospital's security in charge to look into the matter. The security refused to help him saying there was already a warning sign on parking outside the hospital.

The ward boy was heartbroken as the bicycle was new. The chief administrator, showing compassion, took the copy of the ward boy's police report and met the higher management and requested a favour. The hospital management immediately sanctioned the money for a new bicycle. The boy was very happy and thanked the chief administrator. There was resistance from the security in charge, but the management helped the poor boy during the pandemic.

The chief administrator had the courage and will to speak for his staff. Needless to say, the management of most hospitals help staff members in need one way or another.

Income of staff going down during pandemic's first wave

A paramedic was working in the cardiac OPD. Before the pandemic struck, he was working overtime on Sundays to earn ₹5,000 extra, which made it possible to easily pay the EMI on a loan that he had taken. However, the footfall of patients in the OPD came down drastically during the pandemic and during lockdowns, the OPD was closed. As a result, the poor paramedic could not make the extra money by doing overtime and defaulted on paying his EMI.

Doctors and other hospital employees also suffered financially due to the pandemic and lockdown. Many doctors and staff members who had taken bank loans found it difficult to repay them as they were no longer earning as much as they used to before the pandemic. The fear of losing jobs and uncertainty about the pandemic's duration was stressful for both medical and non-medical staff.

Temporary and daily-wage workers, with contractors withholding their wages. Sometimes, such workers left for their native places immediately after receiving their wages. This caused many works in the hospital to remain unfinished.

Unavailability of doctors

Some of the consultants and senior doctors refused to attend to the OPD in spite of repeated reminders. Some of the doctors relented after persuasion by the senior management.

Transportation of employees

The biggest problem was the transportation of staff from their home to the hospital and vice versa. Issues kept on surfacing causing a tough time for administrators. Even when the lockdown was relaxed, the Metro trains didn't start operating, which was a major issue for those employees living far away from the hospital.

Salary deductions

No hospital could have handled the pandemic without the support of the hospital staff. Yet, the hospital management often had no choice but to cut or deduct staff salaries by 15–30 per cent because the hospitals' income also dropped drastically during the pandemic. Some hospitals even terminated the contracts of newly hired staff.

Due to these many problems, the HOD of each department had a tough time motivating their workers, even with all the precautions and the hospital providing treatment to any staff members who were infected.

Reputed hospitals also felt the pressure of the pandemic. In some cases, getting bill payment from the relatives/attendants of a Covid patient who died was next to impossible. Many hospitals waved the outstanding bill amounts in such cases.

Furthermore, during the pandemic each and every employee was afraid their family members may get infected because of them. As a result most of the staff either stayed in the hospital or went home and remained in isolation.

The role of the administrator during the pandemic was not only to counsel their staff to remain positive but also to motivate himself to be strong enough to face these difficulties.

For an administrator, the challenges of saving self and saving hospital staff during the pandemic were enormously difficult to tackle. However, tackling them successfully was vital for keeping the hospital running. And those administrators who rose to the occasion are truly unsung heroes.

Wave II

At the start 2021, lots of activities to control pandemic were initiated. The Union government announced 30,000,000 (three crore) doses of Covaxin – Bharat Biotech's indigenously made anti-Covid-19 vaccine – and Covishield – developed by Oxford University- AstraZeneca and manufactured in India under licence by Serum Institute of India – free of cost for health workers. Apart from this, the government opened thousands of Covid testing and vaccination centres both in public and private hospitals across the country. Citizens could book a slot for the vaccine jab through the government's Aarogya Setu and CoWin apps.

The vaccination drive started from January 16, 2021, in almost all major hospitals and urban health centres throughout the country for people in three phases:

1. For the 60 and above.
2. For the 45 and above
3. For the 18 and above.

Initially, the second dose was planned after 28 days from the first jab, but due to a range of reasons, it was extended to 12 weeks.

After the Wave I ebbed with India recording low Covid-positive cases, life started to get back to pre-pandemic normalcy with schools, offices, and public places, like markets, planning reopening in March.

Then the second phase of the pandemic, referred to as "Wave II", hit the country. It was many times deadlier than the Wave I with new variants of the virus entering the scene. This triggered an unprecedented surge in Covid-19 cases and Covid-related deaths.

Soon, it overwhelmed the already stretched healthcare system in the country. People panicked as hospitals choked with patients and ran out of essential medicines and oxygen.

To tackle the shortage of oxygen, many hospitals installed oxygen plants. They also started additional day-care centres as a stop-gap arrangement just to give oxygen and other care to patients who had breathing difficulties but didn't get a hospital bed.

On top of it, many Covid patients were getting infected with fungi, like black fungus, yellow fungus, and white fungus, which happened for the first time in India. This triggered more panic and caused addition stress to the hospitals.

Hospitals were left with no choice but to turn around countless patients with Covid symptoms by just giving them first aid and day care. Then the Union government announced a new lockdown, in which the conditions were more relaxed than the one imposed during Wave I. This time, the lockdown was of short duration and were reviewed for relaxation every week.

Now, the hospitals started to face new challenges. During Wave II, the hospital administrator had to manage the additional pressure on the following departments:

1. **Security department**: Footfalls increased manyfold with patients, people coming for tests were much higher in numbers than during Wave I.

2. **Parking department:** People coming for getting a vaccine jab or tests came in their own vehicles. *[Note: There was no vaccination going on during Wave I]*

3. **Transport department:** Demand for ambulances and hearses increased manyfold during Wave II as the rate of infection and deaths due to Covid-19 were much higher.

4. **Housekeeping department:** With hospitals getting choked with patients, the department had to work tirelessly with less-than-usual manpower.

5. **Laboratory & diagnostics department:** People coming for tests, like HRCT, increased manyfold. Earlier, it used to take 15–20 minutes to do an HRCT test, but during the Wave II, it took 2–3 hours, or even more, because of the long queues.

Apart from the challenges the above departments faced, imagine the what the doctors and nurses might have gone through while treating patients. They had to wear PPE and work for long hours.

To save the life of patients, both medicos and non-medicos risked their own lives during Wave II.

As Wave II rapidly turned into a nationwide crisis, many hospitals had to take some innovative measures.

Some innovative steps hospitals took during Wave II were:

1. Involved all marketing and corporate staff to assist managers in ward, OPD, IPD, ICU, casualty area, blood bank, etc.

2. Many hospitals restored the pre-pandemic salaries and wages to staff, including doctors and nurses, which were subjected to cuts.

3. The kitchen department in some hospitals provided hot herbal soups (*kadha*) to the hospital staff in the mornings and evenings to keep them fit and energetic.

Some innovations hospital administrators adopted during Wave II:

Wave II was deadlier than Wave I of the pandemic. During Wave II, many new variants of the original Covid-19 virus, which were more contagious and lethal, started infecting people, including the young. Many succumbed to the virus despite getting the best treatment available.

Some hospitals realized that it was important to allow meetings between an admitted patient and his/her family members and friends. Therefore, they set guidelines for the security department to allow such visitors in during visiting hours. The guidelines included wearing of PPE and following the Covid-prevention protocols strictly.

This ensured a dramatic drop in patient side-hospital friction and other patent-side grievances. Apart from this to the surprise of those hospitals, patients started recovering faster!

Government surveillance of hospitals

During the Wave II, the Union government and some state governments kept private hospitals under surveillance for the first time in the history of India. This was a result of many patients and their families complained of several issues, which the media highlighted very prominently.

The Union and state governments took the following measures:

1. Fixed ambulance and hearse charges.

2. Made mandatory that procurement of critical medicines, like remdesivir, anti-fungal drugs, etc, must be from a government agency.

3. Launched a complaint cell to address grievances, like exorbitant hospital bills in Covid-19 treatment.

4. Announced that small children whose both parents died of Covid-19 will get financial support for higher studies after they turn 18.

5. Audited oxygen plants in hospitals for the first time in India.

Apart from the above measures that the Union government took, the Supreme Court also got involved in how the pandemic was handled in the country.

Conclusion:

Doctors and frontline health workers, along with non-medical hospital staff joined hands to fight and defeat the deadly but invisible enemy despite facing every imaginable difficulty. Without their collective effort, Wave II couldn't have been contained.

Lesson 5B

Issues with communication and public relations

I have found that all hospital administrators face unique problems when dealing with:

a.   A large number of calls from outside.

b.   A high number of visitors.

Sometimes, callers calling the hospital to inquire or get an update of an admitted patient don't know the patient's details, which may even include the patient's name, and then start to ask for the same from his associates. At times, callers flaunt their political connections to get discounts or demand "proper treatment", which the hospital always strives to give as its basic duty. In such situations, the administrator must listen carefully and reply courteously to ensure all problems are solved.

Most of the people who call to inquire about patients are:

a.   Family and friends.

b.   Known to hospital owners, doctors, management, representatives, staff, etc.

c.   Local police, government officials, journalists, etc.

d.   Others

A hospital administrator faces other kinds of issues as well, like the following:

a.   Pressure from a patient's relatives for issuing additional visitor passes.

b.   Clash of egos between security staff and patients and/or their attendant, which may lead to quarrels and heated arguments.

To overcome such situations, reputed hospitals have created the following administrative mechanisms:

a. For VVIP patients, the hospital administrator makes arrangements to issue health bulletins to avoid a large number of visitors and/or calls.

b. Most of the hospital authorities, administrators, senior doctors have created groups on social media, like WhatsApp, to address any query without disrupting the hospital's functioning.

c. To tackle local politicians and their entourage who come to the hospital to inquire about the status of the former's relatives or people they know, the administrator coordinates with the relevant departments, doctors, etc, and allows the main person to meet the patient and the treating consultant by making proper arrangements.

d. Sometimes doctors from foreign countries call to learn about a treatment given to a patient or learn the current status of a patient. In such cases, the administrator helps them by giving a fixed time for them to access the on-duty doctors.

e. If a patient's attendant requests, a patient's case summary is provided through email or document-sharing apps, like WhatsApp.

f. If the hospital policy allows, the hospital administrator arranges for a video call between a patient's treating consultant and his relatives.

g. Other miscellaneous mechanisms.

Conclusion: In spite of consultants briefing patients' attendants on the current status of patients during morning and evening rounds, some attendants still seek to leverage their powerful contacts to ensure that the hospital renders "extra care" to the patients. This can cause a higher number of calls and visitors, which may require administrative intervention.

Needless to say, all patients are equal in the eyes of doctors. Hospital management doesn't discriminate on the basis of caste, creed, religion and status.

From past experience as an administrator, I have observed that those who persistently inquire about a patient's treatment and health status and ask more questions are "potential troublemakers". Hence, the administrator needs to be proactive and take all necessary steps to arrange counselling, meetings with treating consultants, etc.

The administrator must maintain his composure all the time and always reply to the queries of patients and attendants courteously. When required, show compassion and try to boost their morale.

"An administrator must have the temperament to assess a situation and react accordingly. He must have good communication skills to put the hospital's point of view firmly without upsetting an attendant or a relative." – VBJ

Lesson 5C

Importance of training and boosting the confidence of housekeeping staff

As I have already mentioned in this book, the hospital's housekeeping department is the backbone of the hospital. This department handles all waste, whether biomedical or normal. This department is also responsible for handing over a deceased patient's body to his/her attendant/relatives.

In all major hospitals, the housekeeping staff keep on bringing things to the notice of the management, like having found something like an ID card, keys, spectacles, money, bag, mobile, shoes, clothes, jewellery, credit cards, health insurance cards, etc, which they find while cleaning the floors. This is all because good training was imparted to them during their induction programme. They were trained to be honest, sincere, hardworking and loyal, and to follow the SOPs. It is always worthwhile to reward and praise employees for doing their work well to boost their confidence and give them more initiative to work diligently.

Let us discuss an imaginary unique incident to highlight this.

Incident:

Once, a patient was brought by his daughter to the emergency department. Immediately, code blue was announced and the patient was put on life support. In the meantime, his daughter had admitted him under TPA billing. In spite of the best medical treatment, the patient expired three days later. His body was kept in the mortuary. The housekeeping staff handed over the mortuary slip to his daughter and the bill was sent to TPA for final approval.

Within two hours, the bill was approved with the addition of certain co-payments along with the differences in the actual bill and the TPA allocation. Then, a man from the deceased side came and asked for the bill, and made the full payment. He was provided with all the papers, including the hospital's death certificate. The man then took all the papers and went to the mortuary area to collect the deceased patient's body.

The housekeeping staff asked for the mortuary slip, which the man did not have, but he insisted on being given the dead body, nevertheless. The housekeeping staff briefed their superiors, who reported to the billing department, who in turn informed the administrator. The administrator came to speak to the man, but also called the girl with the mortuary slip.

The moment the girl came, both she and the gentleman started quarrelling and shouting at each other. Sensing trouble, the administrator called the police who took both of them to the police station and after two hours both were able to come to a mutual solution in writing that the girl would take the death certificate and all the documents, but she would hand over the death certificate and the body to the man.

Because of the housekeeping staff's alertness, the hospital was saved from unnecessary embarrassment. If they had given the body to the man without informing the girl, it would have been a very difficult issue for the hospital management to handle.

Reason that caused the row between the woman and the man:

The deceased patient had two wives who belonged to two different faiths – say Religion A and Religion B. The patient belonged to Religion A, but his name didn't indicate so. The man who paid the outstanding amount in the bill for the deceased patient was the deceased patient's son from his wife, who belonged to Religion A. The woman who collected the deceased patient's documents along with the mortuary slip was the deceased patient's daughter from his other wife, who belonged to Religion B. The woman had admitted him to her office TPA and the entire story has not been told to the billing department. The man and the woman were step-siblings and they both visited the patient regularly that even the ward manager or the billing department which handled the TPA couldn't imagine that such an issue could ever arise.

Words of caution:

1. At the time of discharge, all billing executives must see who admitted the patient for treatment and the billing department must contact the person who signed the admission forms during admission. Even if someone else makes a payment, the documents of a patient (or in case

of death, the body) should be handed over to the person who initially admitted the patient/legal heir.

2. If the patient is conscious and strong enough to handle themselves, there is no problem. But if they are newborn, below 12 years of age, unconscious, drowsy, elderly or are unknown (having been admitted by unknown people), strict protocol must be followed and things, such as ID proof, relation to the patient must be obtained and confirmed, to avoid any problems later on.

3. If a patient expires, the hospital must strictly follow the SOPs of the billing and mortuary departments. All the documents must be carefully checked at each stage of billing. Proper ID proof is mandatory during the handing over of the dead body to the legal heir. The death certificate and mortuary slip must be given to the person who has admitted the patient or the legal heir.

4. The housekeeping supervisor must show the body of a deceased patient to the attendant and check all the documents before giving the body to the deceased's legal heir.

5. MLC bodies must be handed over to the police for postmortem purposes.

6. The administrator also faces the problem where an expired patient's relative wants to donate the eye, organ or even the entire dead body according to the last wishes of the deceased. Again, SOPs must be followed strictly, including the legal heir's request. Whenever such problems arise, senior management must be present to supervise everything until the body leaves the hospital.

7. Other checks and verifications.

"Handling death cases is a very sensitive issue. Always ensure proper documentation and follow SOPs and checklists before handing over documents and body to the legal heir so that the hospital can avoid liabilities in the future." – VBJ

Lesson 6

Final words from the hospital administrator

The hospital administrator is the goodwill ambassador of the hospital. In most cases, it has been seen that both clinical and non-clinical issues lead to administrative problems. Hence all three important pillars of the hospital: the medical superintendent, chief administrator, and nursing superintendent are responsible for solving these administrative issues.

All the above administrators are specialized in their field of work, which they use to ensure the following things for the patient:

a. Treatment

b. Nursing care

c. Safety

d. Well-being and satisfaction.

Word-of-mouth promotion by patients, attendants and their relatives are the main source for the growth and success of hospitals. The three administrative pillars must always contribute their 100 per cent to build the hospital's brand, which the marketing department always advertises.

The administrator plays a vital role and works in two ways:

a. At the staff's level.

b. At the patient's or their attendant's level.

At staff level:

All hospital staff responsible for handling the treatment of a patient irrespective of which part/department of the hospital they work in. They must fully comply with the standard operating procedures.

At patient's or their attendant's level

The hospital administrator ensures that:

1. A patient's treatment is done according to medical guidelines.

2. The laboratory & diagnostics reports and the procedures done on patients must be accurate and correct.

3. All the departments meet the hospital's standards.

4. The food served to patients is safe, nutritious, and hygienic.

5. Medicines at the pharmacy are genuine and bills are provided for each transaction.

6. The family and attendant of a patient have the right to be kept updated on the health and the prognosis of the patient.

To ensure the hospital's growth and upgradation, the following policies should be maintained:

a. **Mission policy** – For example, to provide healthcare services through qualified and experienced professionals with a patient-friendly attitude.

b. **Vision policy** – For example, to achieve excellence through constant upgrades to the facility and the training of the staff.

c. **Quality policy** – For example, to Ensure that the system is free of defects.

If the above policies are implemented, then it will be easy for the organization to achieve its objectives, which is primarily to build a strong brand for the hospital and growth of the hospital.

Thoughts for policymakers:

To recognize the invaluable contribution of non-medicos in the healthcare sector, there should be a day dedicated to commemorate them. There should be a "Non-Medicos' Day", just like Doctors' Day and Nurses' Day, to honour the tireless work of non-medical staff in hospitals, like the administrators, managers, billing staff, maintenance staff, housekeeping staff, security staff, transport staff, etc. Without them, the healthcare sector can't function.

There should be discussions, seminars, etc, on how the medical and the non-medical staff should complement each other in keeping the healthcare sector running.

Final message from the veteran administrator to the upcoming administrators:

1. Administrators must develop a basic mechanism to help them in managing the hospital, such as the **A**, **B**, **C** of administration:

   a. **Anticipation** – they must anticipate problems.

   b. **Believe** – they must believe in the facts.

   c. **Consequences** – they should be able to foresee the consequences of a situation in advance so that their negative impact can be minimized.

A smart administrator must respond quickly without wasting time, know the value of the customer's (patient's) trust and be proactive in solving issues.

"Avoiding an unpleasant situation is better than firefighting after an untoward incident has happened. React quickly and look for solutions to resolve a problem or an issue before it gets out of hands."– VBJ

---

2. Hospitals must be system-driven with implementation of SOPs and not man-driven. Keeping things transparent will ensure professional competence, business ethics, lesser problems and maximum benefits.

"Learning is a continuous process, hence always be on the quest to better even the best." – VBJ

References

1. Economic Survey 2019-20, Volume -2, Government of India, Ministry of Finance, Department of Economic Affairs, North Block, New Delhi – 110001.

2. Kailash Hospital Policies, Version 5 (released on December 2017). The Kailash Hospital is a unit of Kailash Healthcare Limited and is located at H-33, Sector 27, Noida, District Gautam Buddh Nagar, Uttar Pradesh – 201301 Noida.

Acknowledgement

I am thankful to following people, which include my seniors, doctors, nurses, paramedics, technicians, patients, children of hospital staff, friends, and others. Without their inputs, insights and motivation, this book would not have been possible. Some of the noteworthy names are:

- Dr Vijay Ganju, medical superintendent

- Mrs E.O. Mariamma, Metron

- Mrs Sunita Masih, chief administrator

- Mr Sambhu Nath Dubey, administrator

- Mrs Poonam Singh, administrator

- Ms Richa Pandey, assistant professor, MBA Healthcare and Hospital Administration, Sharda University

- Ms Dimple Eleazer (Administrator)

- Mrs Anita Tiwari, OPD administrator

- Mrs Tannu Sharma, OPD administrator

- Mrs Supriya Trivedi, casualty manager

- Mrs Puniyan Sharma, Chief PRO

- Mrs Sonika Singh, chief dietician

- Mr Shiv Lal Sharma, CSSD technician

- Mr Ram Mehar, security in charge

- Mrs Sadhna Verma, housekeeping in charge

- Mr Chhote Lal, housekeeping supervisor

- Mr Pankaj Sharma, lawyer

- Mr Bhanu Joshi, Studying Brown University, USA

- Mr Rabin Sebi, hotel management executive

- Mr Vimlesh, computer operator

- Mr Dinesh, office boy

- Mrs Zora Khatoon, patient

This book has been edited by Mr Jayanta Bhattacharya, independent journalist, and proofread by Mr Kaushik Chatterjee, HR consultant.

Glossary

ABG	:	arterial blood gas
ACLS	:	advance cardiac life Support
AF	:	atrial fibrillation
AI	:	artificial intelligence
AMC	:	annual maintenance contract
aya	:	female helpers who do similar work as ward boys
BIPAP	:	bilevel positive airway pressure
BLS	:	basic life support
BP	:	blood pressure
C-section:		caesarean section
CA	:	chartered accountant
CABG	:	coronary artery (bypass) graft/surgery
CAD	:	coronary artery disease
CBC	:	complete blood count
CCMO	:	chief casualty medical officer
CCU	:	coronary care unit
CEO	:	chief executive officer
CGHS	:	Central Government Health Service
COO	:	chief operating officer
COPD	:	chronic obstructive pulmonary disease
CPR	:	cardiopulmonary resuscitation
CRF	:	chronic renal failure
CT scan:		computerized tomography.
CTVS	:	cardiothoracic and vascular surgery

CVA	:	cerebrovascular accident
CXR	:	chest x-ray
DM	:	diabetic mellitus
DOR	:	discharge on request
Dr	:	doctor
ECG	:	electrocardiogram
ECHS	:	Ex-Servicemen Contributory Health Scheme
EEG	:	electroencephalography
ENT	:	ear, nose, and throat
FBS	:	fasting blood sugar
FMCG	:	fast-moving consumer goods
GIPSA	:	General Insurance Public Sector Association
Gurudakshina:		The tradition of repaying one's teacher after the completion of formal training/education
Hb	:	haemog lobin
HbA1C:		test to measure the amount of blood sugar attached to haemoglobin
HDU	:	high-dependency unit
HIV	:	human immunodeficiency virus
HTN	:	hypertension
ICU	:	intensive care unit
IT	:	information technology
IU	:	international unit
IV	:	intravenous
KFT	:	kidney function test
LAMA	:	leave against medical advice
LFT	:	liver function test
MI	:	myocardial infraction
MICU	:	medical intensive care unit

MLC	:	medico-legal case
MRD	:	medical record department
MRI	:	magnetic resonance imaging
NEFT	:	National Electronic Funds Transfer
NPO	:	nil par os (nothing by mouth)
OPD	:	outpatient department
OT	:	operation theatre
RBC	:	red blood cell
RMO	:	resident medical officer
RTA	:	road traffic accident
RTGS	:	real-time gross settlement
SOS	:	save our souls (if needed/in emergency)
TPA	:	third-party administrator
USG	:	ultrasonography
VBJ	:	Vishwa Bandhu Joshi (the author of this book)
VIP	:	very important person
VVIP	:	very, very important person